SAFER CARE

Human Factors for Healthcare

COURSE HANDBOOK

Edited by Patrick Mitchell

Prepared on behalf of the North East Strategic Health Authority Patient Safety Action Team

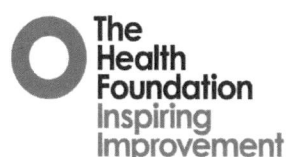
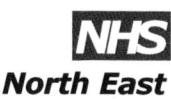
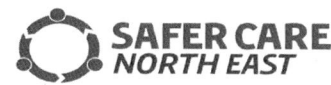

Safer Care—Human Factors in Healthcare: Course Handbook
Edited by Patrick Mitchell

First published 2013
ISBN: 978-1-909675-01-8
Copyright © 2013 Swan & Horn
All rights reserved.

No part of this publication may be reproduced, stored in a retrieval system, or transmitted in any form or by any means, electronic, mechanical, photocopying, recording or otherwise, without either the prior permission of the publisher on behalf of the NHS Commissioning Board, or a licence permitting restricted copying in the United Kingdom issued by the Copyright Licensing Agency, 90 Tottenham Court Road, London, W1T 4LP — except in the case of brief quotations embodied in critical reviews and certain other noncommercial uses permitted by fair use in copyright law. For permission requests, contact the publisher Swan & Horn, phone: (44) 1436 842749, fax: 07092 373804 or email: info@swanandhorn.co.uk.

Any person who does any unauthorised act in relation to this publication may be liable to criminal prosecution and civil claims for damages.

Notice
Clinical practice is constantly evolving in terms of standard safety precautions, responsibility of practitioners and treatment options. While every effort has been made to ensure the accuracy of information contained in this publication, no guarantee can be given that all errors and omissions have been excluded. Neither the publisher nor the authors assume any liability for any injury and/or damage to persons or property arising from this publication.

The Publisher
For information and orders, contact Swan & Horn:
Swan & Horn • Woodside Tower •
Cove • Argyll and Bute G84 0NT
Tel: (44)1436 842748 • Fax: 07092 373804
Email: info@swanandhorn.co.uk
www.swanandhorn.co.uk

Cover artwork by Virginia Brailsford
Editorial and production by Shoreline BioMedical
Printed in England by Ferguson Print, Keswick

Contents

Preface — *iii*
Contributors — *v*

Introduction — *vii*
List of Figures — *xi*

LEARNING MODULES

1	Thinking About Thinking—Cognitive Processing	1–13
2	Decision Making	15–26
3	Situation Awareness	27–38
4	Personality Type	39–50
5	Team Working	51–62
6	Leadership	63–74
7	Communication	75–91
8	Stress and Fatigue	93–106

Index — 107–115

With special thanks to:
Professor Graham Towl, Professor David Crighton
and Durham University Department of Psychology

Preface

Safer Care is a training course on human factors for all healthcare professionals. It was developed by the Safer Care Action Team, NHS North East of England, and consists of eight modules dealing with cognitive processing, decision-making, situation awareness, personality types, teamwork, leadership, communication skills, and stress management. This *Handbook* gives detailed accounts of each of these subjects and can be used in conjuction with the e-learning package at www.safercare.eu/human/.

Human factors training is widely used in safety-critical industries, but healthcare is a relative latecomer to the field. There are two main differences from other industries that must be addressed. The first, and more obvious, one relates to those issues that are specific to healthcare, as opposed to those of primary relevance to other industries.

The second is less obvious, but more important. It relates to the fact that healthcare professionals tend to be more sceptical than workers in many other industries – they are disinclined to accept statements of benefit without seeing the evidence. This course has been specially designed with this important difference in mind.

Contributors

CLIVE BLOXHAM
Clive Bloxham is a consultant pathologist at County Durham and Darlington Hospitals with an interest in cognitive factors in medical practice and how errors occur.

GUY HIRST
Guy Hirst was a pilot with British Airways from 1972 until 2006 and was one of the pioneers of Human Factors Training in the airline culture. Since 2001 he has been writing and presenting courses in healthcare and is involved in research on healthcare safety.

PHIL LAWS
Phil Laws is a consultant in intensive care medicine and anaesthesia in Newcastle, and medical lead for the Advanced Critical Care Practitioner Programme and Outreach, with an interest in communication, crisis communication for junior doctors and mandatory training for critical care staff.

PATRICK MITCHELL
Patrick Mitchell is a consultant neurosurgeon in Newcastle upon Tyne with a research interest in surgical safety and decision-making.

EMMA NUNEZ
Emma Nunez is a registered midwife who now works in patient safety. She is the Safer Care North East Programme manager and chaired the Human Factors Faculty responsible for developing this course.

NANCY REDFERN
Nancy Redfern is a consultant anaesthetist in Newcastle upon Tyne specialising in obstetric and neuro-anaesthesia, with an interest in medical education, appraisal and mentorship.

GAVIN THOMS
Gavin Thom is a consultant anaesthetist with interests in perioperative and operative safety, and related human and cultural factors. He is currently joint lead on Project OASIS on surgical safety in South East Asia and recently led the international Global Oximetry Project aimed at improving anaesthetic safety.

Introduction

Being human, by its very nature, makes us all fallible. The additional titles we bear – doctor, nurse, midwife, pharmacist, dentist, chief executive, non-executive director (the list is endless) as a result of our education, training and technical ability – will never change the fundamental imperfections found among humans.

Our day-to-day lives provide numerous opportunities to make mistakes that generally have limited adverse consequences. You might forget to put the bin out on collection day because of some distraction, or you might walk down the stairs with the intention of emptying the washing machine, only to forget what you came down for when you reach the kitchen. These lapses are only minor, no more than an irritation, meaning that you have to make alternative plans for refuse disposal or you have to stop in your tracks and retrace your steps to work out what it was you had meant to do. These kind of mistakes do not harm anyone.

However, some lapses carry greater risks. A midwife, for example, driving home in the early hours after finishing her nightshift, pulled to a stop at a red traffic light. As she sat and waited for the lights to change, the CD she was playing came to the end and the player automatically changed to the next disc in the library. At this point she drove off again, right through the red light. She had confused the change in what she heard with the change she was waiting to see in the traffic signals. She laughed about it at the time, but she was well aware of how easily she could have killed or seriously injured herself or someone else.

Let us not make the error of thinking that the processes we experience that lead to mistakes in our personal and social lives are any different from the processes we experience that lead to mistakes in our professional life. Why do we tend to think that the title of our professional group removes our fallibility? Why is it that we forget such risks when it comes to delivering some of the most technologically advanced and effective healthcare in the world? What has led us to think this way?

When we talk about improving safety and reliability in healthcare, we make regular references to the aviation industry. The aviation industry has considerable knowledge and learning that can be shared with and applied to healthcare, but the industry embarked on a difficult journey when it first introduced human factors training. The following quote is from Jeremy Butler, the General Manager of Flight Training in British Airways at that time. We thank him for allowing us to use his comments here, which reveal a rational, balanced view based on both his own experience and expertise in aviation, and latterly in healthcare.

> *"Flight Ops in British Airways (BA) had for a few years been considering, rather idly, the issues of what we might now call non-technical skills on the flight deck. I had become interested in Human Factors, both at the managerial and front-line levels, and became informed through attending seminars and conferences in the USA. I participated in the United Airlines CRM programme (called something else but I can't remember the exact name). I was asked by*

Introduction

Operating Standards Group (OSG) in BA whether this had any relevance to us. I enjoyed the experience but it was a very psychological course at that time, and I concluded that British pilots were not ready for 'psychobabble'. Also I believed that the Standard Operating Procedures of BA were greatly superior to those of the manufacturer, which are usually adopted by airline operators. It seemed to me that the principles of the 'monitored approach' with workload distribution and shared responsibilities were conducive to achieving safe flight and that Crew Resource Management (CRM) was not necessary in BA.

"I believe the Kegworth accident changed the thinking in BA (there was probably active consideration prior to Kegworth, and this confirmed the thinking, but I can't remember the exact sequence). The Board Air Safety Committee (not sure of the exact name now), decided that we would develop and introduce a CRM programme. The responsibility for this fell to me. This was devolved to various managers and interested flight crew, and we recruited a number of CRM instructors. It is noteworthy that CRM was introduced in BA well before the Civil Aviation Authority (CAA) had made it a requirement (even though it was hugely expensive). I have always believed that leading world operators have a responsibility to be generative and not simply respond to the Regulatory Authority. This is an example of BA leading in the UK and influencing the Authority as well as other airlines worldwide.

"At some point (1992, I think) I became Chair of International Air Transport Association (IATA) Human Factors Group and worked with Dan Maurino in International Civil Aviation Organisation (ICAO) and we took Human Factors/CRM to the world's airlines!"

Jeremy has also worked in several different roles within the NHS, which have allowed him to reflect on the years he spent in aviation.

"During my time working in the NHS, I have also pondered why the messages so obvious to us were not being universally received. I am now working with a NHS Research and Ethics Committee and a member of the National Research Ethics Advisors' Panel. This new insight has demonstrated something of which I was certainly aware, but not in so dominant a fashion, and that is that the medical profession will not do anything without evidence. In healthcare this evidence is accrued over many years of research studies, perhaps in some cases (a very few) resulting in new treatments or new medications. This evidence base is the safety mechanism of healthcare, and I support it. In aviation, I fear that we have not gathered in sufficient detail or depth the evidence for human factors/ CRM interventions as a necessary component in improving safety. I introduced CRM to BA on an instinctive feel, after attending conferences and seminars in the USA, but with very little research or analysis and no idea of how to measure outcomes of safety improvement. Of course we struggle with these measures as the data is very limited. Do you remember 'Cockpit 2000', a highly controversial component of our CRM programme? I thought it seemed a good idea at the time, and to this day I have no idea of its worth, although I am aware of the aggro.

"All this preamble is to say that we, involved in aviation human factors, have been remiss in not acquiring and documenting the evidence that HF and CRM have improved aviation safety. We should have been measuring the effects of our interventions, doing genuine research and writing learned articles in Aerospace for years, but we haven't. Is it too late to start? I don't know, as I am not closely involved anymore, but I am sure that the medical profession will continue to ask 'What is the evidence?'"

Introduction

These intimate reflections on both the aviation and healthcare industries reinforce the question *why are we not doing this already?* Professionals from other high-risk industries are often stunned to learn that this is not already a part of our mandatory professional education and progression; they assume that "clinical" human factors must be an intrinsic part of how we train.

This is not the place for a debate on the definition of "clinical human factors' – there are many other places where such a debate is on-going. However, the fact that we are even talking about the subject in the context of delivering healthcare is a positive step forward. The aim of this book and course, therefore, is to support the individuals and teams involved in delivery of healthcare, to understand the connection between the "psychobabble" surrounding the analysis of the human mind, and what it means to you in practice. It explains how cognition (the process of how we "think"), decision making, situation awareness (our view of what is happening around us), our personalities and their differences, team working, leadership, communication skills, and stress and fatigue apply to us when we are providing care and treatment to patients. Perhaps more importantly, it enhances understanding of these factors and therefore assists us in delivering care and treatment safely.

Many have argued that we cannot apply all the information gained from the aviation industry to healthcare, saying *I don't deal with planes. I deal with patients!* Is this not an even stronger argument for the need to understand human factors within healthcare? We cannot programme patients, or their disease, injury or illness, but we can avoid deluding ourselves that our years of technical training and experience remove our vulnerability as humans. We are, after all, "only human".

EMMA NUNEZ

List of Figures

Figure 1.1	Triggers to switch between automatic and analytic thinking	6
Figure 1.2	Factors influencing transition between automatic and analytic thinking	7
Figure 1.3	The unconscious thought theory	11
Figure 2.1	The options check	16
Figure 2.2	Graph of unconscious thought theory showing the effect of quality and complexity of a situation on thought	25
Figure 3.1	The situation awareness (SA) check	30
Figure 3.2	The three levels of situation awareness (SA)	34
Figure 3.3	Examples of the cards used in Asch's group conformity experiments	35
Figure 4.1	A woodcut depicting the four classical temperaments	40
Figure 4.2	Carl Jung's model of personality	42
Figure 5.1	The Swiss cheese model	58
Figure 5.2	The University of Texas Threat and Error Management (TEM) model	60
Figure 6.1	Key attributes of effective leaders in the NHS	74
Figure 7.1	SMRC communication model and feedback	76
Figure 7.2	Equipment needed for intubation (structured version)	79
Figure 7.3	Equipment needed for intubation (narrative version)	81
Figure 8.1	The Yerkes–Dodson relationship between stimulus strength and visual discrimination and learning in mice (published in 1908) and the stylised version as found in the popular psychology press	99
Figure 8.2	Matrix of different conflict management strategies and performance and satisfaction in teams	101
Figure 8.3	Typical PTSD reactions to trauma at different times after the initial trauma	103

Thinking About Thinking: Cognitive Processing

Key points for reflection

❶ We all have biases in our cognitive processing that will influence decision-making. For example, evidence that supports what we already think is more readily attended to than evidence that contradicts it.

❷ We must learn to distinguish between automatic and unconscious thinking and actions, and analytic and conscious thinking and actions.

❸ We should recognise biases in our cognitive processes and adjust accordingly for these where appropriate.

The word "cognition" means mental information processing of conscious and unconscious thought. It has been estimated that 70% of medical errors are due to faulty cognition. In clinical judgement and decision-making, results suggests that habits of thought are skills that are as important as traditional diagnostic and procedural skills, and they are open to refinement and improvement with training.

The Dual Process Model

Current psychology uses a dual process mode.

Vignette 1.1 Dual Process Model—Example 1

An early modern human some tens of thousands of years ago, is applying analytic thought to lighting a fire. When a wild animal approaches, he switches to automatic to escape.

Vignette 1.2 Dual Process Model—Example 2

A surgeon doing a cholecystectomy is largely in automatic mode while applying analytic thinking to discussions in the theatre. When heavy bleeding starts, analytic thinking is suddenly directed to the operation.

Table 1.1 *The Dual Process Model*

Property	Automatic (System 1)	Analytic (System 2)
Reasoning style	Intuitive, heuristic, associative, concrete	Conscious, normative, deductive, abstract
Working memory	Not involved	Involved
Awareness	Low	High
Action	Reflexive, skilled	Deliberate, rule-based
Automaticity	High	Low
Speed	Fast	Slow
Effort	Minimal	Considerable
Cost	Low	High
Vulnerability to bias	Yes	Less so
Reliability	Low, variable	High, consistent
Errors	Common	Few
Predictive power	Low	High
Hard-wired	May be	No
Scientific rigour	Low	High
Context importance	High	Low

Which system is best?

Neither is better than the other. The automatic system gets a bad press for being primitive and being less flexible than the analytic system, but it is much faster, and when engaged appropriately, it is more accurate. Both have been conserved in human evolution and have equally valuable roles in reasoning.

Automatic cognition

Heuristics are rules that automatic cognitive processes follow. They are not rules of the explicit kind such as "look both ways before crossing the road", but take the form of deep *tacit knowledge* that is not easily formulated or told to others.

They are information-processing shortcuts learned from experience, and are sometimes called cognitive *rules of thumb*.

We are generally not aware of *using* heuristics, only of their outcomes. Heuristics are selected by conscious or unconscious pattern recognition; they then determine an individual's further action.

These scenarios illustrate two modes of thinking – *automatic* and *analytic* – and how these modes have been highly conserved over human evolution. We all have these two modes; of thinking – *the key is to be able to switch between them appropriately.*

There are around fifty know heuristics, a selection of which are shown below, together with their main characteristics.

Table 1.2 *Six common heuristics and their characteristics*

Name of heuristic	Characteristic
Availability	The tendency to judge an event as more likely if it readily comes to mind (e.g. recent exposure to a disease)
Anchoring	The disposition to persist with an initial judgement regardless of new information to the contrary
Confirmation	The tendency to actively seek evidence to support a given position, rather than evidence that might refute it
Representative	Decisions based on recognising a prototype, or "typical" example of a class of diseases without considering base rates or atypical variants
Premature closing	The premature closing of the decision-making process before it has been fully verified
Sutton's slip	The diagnostic approach of going for the obvious without considering alternative possibilities. The name derives from the story of the Brooklyn bank-robber Willie Sutton who when asked by the judge why he robbed banks answered *'Because that's where the money is*!'

Heuristics are also referred to as *cognitive biases* because they determine our preference for drawing one conclusion over another due to psychological factors, rather than objective evidence.

In this situation the word *bias* refers to a normal and usually valuable mental asset. This is automatic heuristic cognition; it is:

- Fast—with no appreciable delay between pattern recognition and guide to further action.
- Requires little mental effort.
- The default mental process (for the two reasons above).

Unlike analytic cognition, automatic cognition appears to operate in multiple, parallel pathways. It may be that its speed allows effective multitasking through a single channel, but the effect is the same.

There are *three* types of error that automatic cognition is particularly prone to – omission, commission and substitution.

> ### Errors associated with automatic cognition
>
> **Errors of omission** occur when something should be done but nothing is, such as missing a check on a checklist because of distraction.
>
> **Errors of commission** occur when nothing should be done but something is, such as the traffic light error described in Introduction.
>
> **Errors of substitution** occur when something should be done but the wrong thing is, such as opening the oven door instead of the fridge door to get some milk.

Things that promote automatic cognition

Automatic cognition is promoted by distracting influences that make it difficult for someone to give a problem the attention that analytic thought requires. These distractions include emotional state, tiredness and fatigue.

Other problems requiring analytic attention such as financial concerns, family matters, and so on, do not impair our ability to switch into analytic thinking mode but do occupy the single and slow analytic channel.

EMOTIONAL STATE

Particularly negative emotions like frustration and anger make it difficult to switch into analytic mode. Successful switching to analytic thought lessens the intensity of such emotions. This is an important part of conflict resolution, where leading an agitated person towards analytic thinking is a valuable strategy.

TIREDNESS AND FATIGUE

Tiredness is a short-term state that is aggravated by sustained concentration, sleep deprivation and stress. Switching to analytic thinking is more difficult when a person is tired. The solution to tiredness is simply a good night's rest.

Fatigue has a similar meaning to tiredness, but is often used to describe a longer-term state that is aggravated by long periods of high-intensity cognitive effort over weeks, cumulative sleep deprivation, and other life stresses. As with tiredness, fatigue reduces our ability to switch to analytic thinking. Common experience suggests that the solution is a holiday rather than the good night's rest (see *Module 8*).

Multiple interruptions

Multiple interruptions have little impact on *automatic* thinking because:

- It is faster than analytic thinking.
- It is largely unconscious.

However, multiple interruptions have a profound effect on *analytic* thinking because:

- The processing speed is slow and therefore more prone to any interruption.
- Analytic thinking is more complex, so an interruption means that more backtracking has to be done to get back to the same point.

Failing to switch from automatic to analytic mode

If we remain in automatic mode when we should switch to analytic, errors can arise. This switch usually happens appropriately, but the risk of failing to switch, or to consciously guide automatic processes, rises with the above factors.

We do not get stuck in automatic, but we can drift by default in an automatic mode of working until we consciously direct such thinking in response to events. Look at **Vignette 1.3** below.

> **Vignette 1.3 Accidental anaesthesia**
>
> After a caesarean section, intravenous co-amoxiclav (an antibiotic) is given to prevent infection.
>
> A woman had a caesarean section under spinal anaesthesia and was cuddling her new baby. The anaesthetist checked with patient and staff for any allergy to antibiotics, then administered the drug over three minutes.
>
> The patient rapidly became unconscious and required emergency intubation and ventilation. She made a full and rapid recovery.
>
> Later it emerged that the drug given was the anaesthetic induction agent, thiopentone, which was drawn up ahead of time in a 20 mL syringe, and is a pale-straw coloured liquid, like the antibiotic.
>
> This was an automatic cognition error of substitution.

Analytic cognition

Analytic cognition is a slow, largely conscious, cognitive process. It consumes more mental effort than automatic thinking and is much more tiring. It is associated with physiological changes, such as a rise in blood pressure and heart rate.

> **Advantages and disadvantages of analytic cognition**
>
> Its great *advantage* over automatic thinking is its flexibility. Automatic thinking depends largely on pattern recognition, and it does not work well when no pattern is recognised (and it is prone to recognising the wrong pattern). Analytic thinking is capable of assessing and avoiding both of these errors.
>
> The *disadvantage* is that unlike automatic thinking it must be positively engaged. We default to automatic mode rather than analytic mode.

For some problems there may be no viable solution from analytic thinking. Craster's well-known poem *Centipede's Dilemma (overpage)* illustrates the limitation of analytic thinking.

> *The centipede was happy—quite!*
> *Until the toad in fun*
> *Said "Pray, which leg comes after which?"*
> *Which brought his mind to such a pitch*
> *He lay distracted in a ditch*
> *Considering how to run.*

Because it is a slow single-channel process, our ability to respond to situations with analytic thought can be impaired if the channel is preoccupied by other matters. Our consciousness is dominated by analytic thinking when we are engaged in it, and the conscious threshold for external stimuli rises. In extreme cases, this situation is known as *fixation*. In fixation, analytic thought is so dominated by one issue that the conscious threshold for sensory inputs is greatly raised, so far that things such as warning sounds or lights or other people speaking are not registered at all. We *drift* into automatic thinking, but in this way we can get *stuck* in analytic thinking.

Switching between automatic and analytic thinking

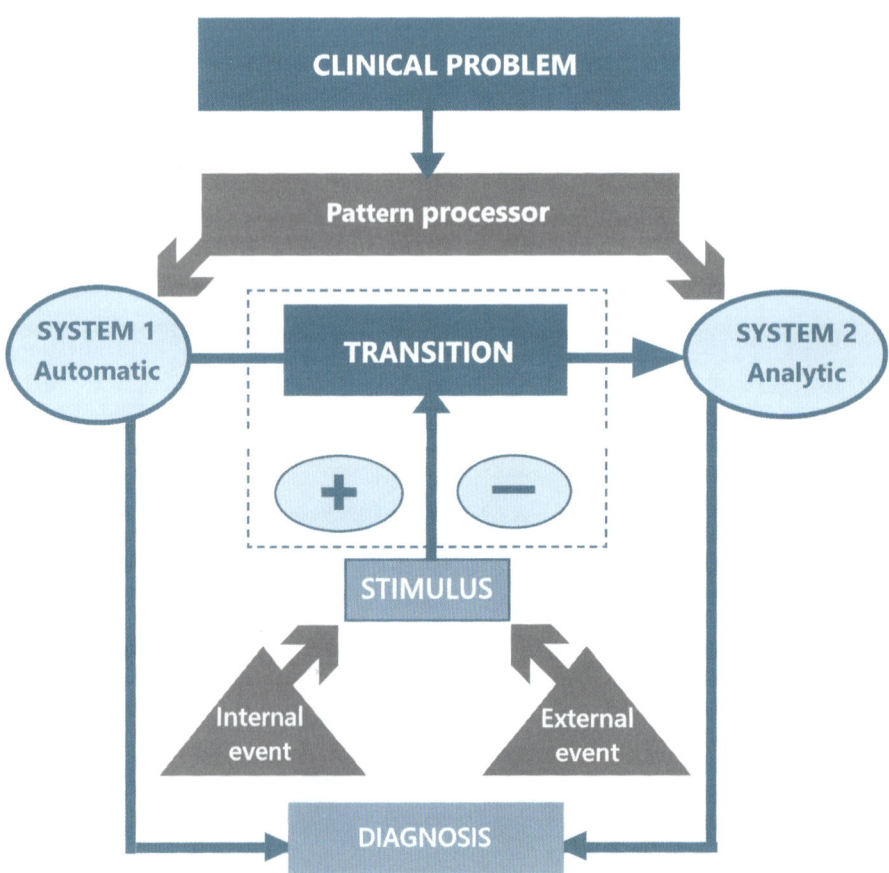

Figure 1.1 *Triggers to switch between automatic and analytic thinking, and factors that promote (+) or retard (-) switching to analytic mode. Triggers can be internal (e.g. an uneasy feeling) or external (e.g. a warning sign). The area outlined by the dashed lines is expanded in Figure 1.2*

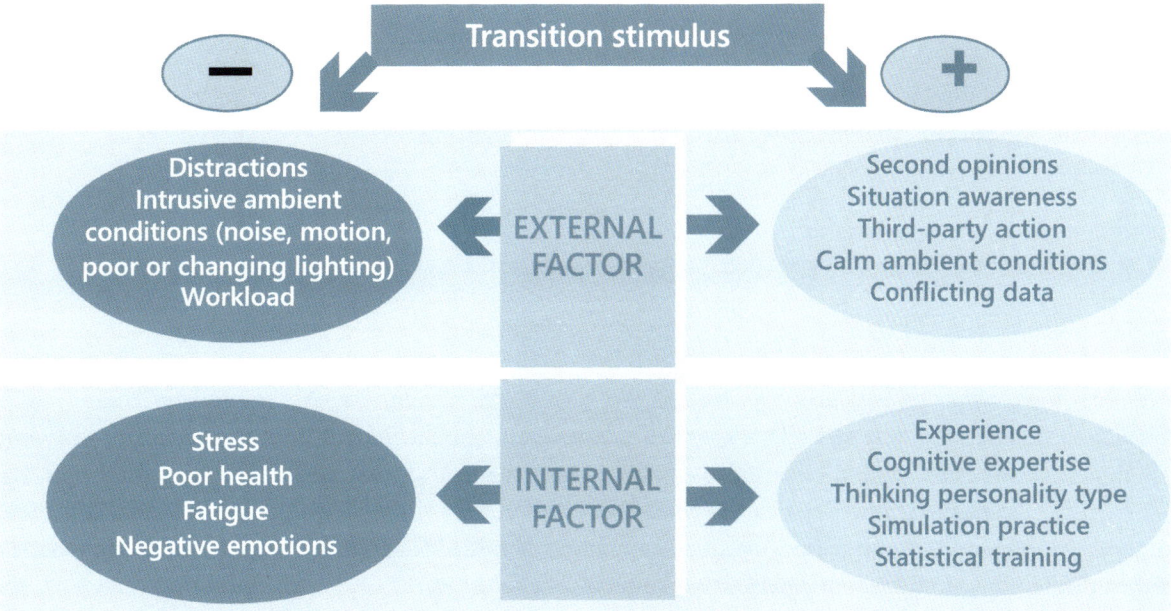

Figure 1.2 *Factors influencing transition between System 1 (automatic) and System 2 (analytic) thinking.*

A selection of the most significant determinants for switching is given in **Figure 1.1** on previous page. Here they are classified according to their source and whether they have a positive or negative influence on the transition process.

Even without the influence of environmental factors and experiences, people will vary in their disposition for automatic versus analytic thinking. For example:

- It depends on the individual's personality and other characteristics, including their Intelligence Quotient (IQ).

- Automatic errors are more likely when there are distractions or time pressures that reduce the attention and effort required for the functioning of conscious analysis.

The nature of the judgement itself influences automatic *versus* analytic thinking:

- Matters such as deciding on what car to buy involve consideration of numerous complex factors and engage analytic thinking.

- Deciding which way to go on a familiar route on your way to work engages automatic thinking.

Whether an issue is dealt with automatically or analytically depends on the way that the information is presented. In **Vignette 1.3**, for example, the syringe of thiopentone looked like co-amoxiclav. This kind of pattern recognition is influenced more by sight, sound, smell and touch than it is by language.

A junior doctor asking his or her consultant about treatment may present a clear and typical history and suggest an appropriate treatment, before asking '*Do you agree?*' The consultant is then likely to say '*Yes*' *automatically*. If there is any ambiguity or inconsistency between the clinical picture and the proposed treatment, the consultant is likely to deal with the case *analytically*. Each response is appropriate to its situation.

Unconscious processing

Ideas about the subconscious mind are polarised between psychoanalytic and psychological theories; different schools from different historical contexts use different methods of evidence gathering.

- Psychoanalysis uses detailed case studies of people undergoing repeated therapy sessions.
- Psychology uses laboratory experiments and data from surveys.

Freud's psychodynamic theory

Freud's theory of mind was an early attempt to explain human behaviour in terms of basic physical and chemical mechanisms *without* recourse to any supernatural effects. It removed the last barrier to viewing humans as physical machines, so dealing what Freud called the *third blow* to the medieval theistic view of the human mind. (The first blow was the cosmological blow of Copernicus who ended the geocentric view of the universe; the second was Darwin's theory of evolution.)

Freud saw the mind as an *energy system*, in which mental content is not simply stored but exerts pressure on behaviour. Psychodynamic theory concerns the source of that energy, how it flows, gets side-tracked, becomes dammed up, and is expressed.

> **The essential features of Freud's theory**
>
> ■ Mental energy is strictly limited, and energy used for one purpose is not available for another.
>
> ■ Mental energy is conserved so that if it is blocked from expression in one channel it becomes diverted inevitably into another (rather than disappearing).
>
> ■ The mind operates to relieve tension created by bodily needs, thus a shortage of food leads to a tension called 'hunger' which is eliminated in the mind by seeking environmental factors that mitigate hunger (namely food), thereby achieving quiescence.
>
> ■ All behaviour is directed towards achieving pleasure, either by reducing tension or by releasing energy.
>
> *Note that these processes are largely unconscious.*

Freud also proposed three different levels of awareness of mental processes:

- **Conscious**—At this level are thoughts that we are aware of at the time that we are having them. This is still the definition used for the content of consciousness.

- **Preconscious**—These are thoughts and memories that we are not conscious of at the time we are having them, but could easily become aware of if we attended to them (such as your own birth date or home address, or the outline and progress of a project you are involved with).

- **Unconscious**—At this level are things that we cannot become aware of except under specific circumstances, such as slips of the tongue, neuroses, works of art, psychosis and dreams. They are suppressed because they cause stress. These unconscious processes have a profound effect on conscious thought and behaviour.

Freud based his unconscious levels on evidence gained from clinical hypnosis. If a person is asked to remember something while hypnotised, when they are woken up they cannot remember it and do not know that they have forgotten it. However, when they are hypnotised again, they often remember it. This shows that the information must have been stored unconsciously.

Id, ego and superego

Freud added to his three-tiered theory of consciousness in 1923 with the concepts of the *id*, *ego* and *superego*.

> - **The id**—This was proposed as the source of all mental energy. Its purpose is to reduce tension arising from biological drivers to return to a peaceful mental state. It does this by seeking pleasure and avoiding pain. The id is entirely unconscious, and entirely uncomplicated. It does not plan or temporise, but merely seeks immediate pleasure or release of tension. It has a tenuous link to the physical world and can be satisfied by imagination as well as action.
>
> - **The superego**—The superego represents the learnt moral aspects of social behaviour, including standards of ethics and conduct. It is largely unconscious and has a limited ability to interact with the external world.
>
> - **The ego**—The ego is the principle constituent of consciousness and stands between the id and the superego. It directly controls conscious thought and actions, moderating the demands of the id and superego according to what is reasonable and achievable in practice. Unlike the id and superego, however, the ego has the ability to plan, to weigh options and to temporise.

Freud's theory is one of an unconscious cauldron of motivational tensions and mental energy. These can be controlled and redirected, but they must be manifested, sometimes in ways apparently unrelated to their origin (such as irrational beliefs or psychosomatic illness).

Experimental evidence of unconscious processes

In 1884, a group of researchers investigated their own abilities to distinguish between differing weights. They plotted their confidence in the difference between these weights against the accuracy of their judgements and found that even when they had no confidence at all that the weights were different, their "pure guesses" were still correct 60% of the time. This finding was of high statistical significance.

In the 1960s and 1970s, experiments on what we now call *subliminal perception* confirmed that the threshold for unconscious registration of information is lower than the threshold for *conscious* registration – for all sensory modalities. This threshold can be in terms of the duration the information is presented for, or of the level of intensity at which it is presented. The threshold varies with the factors listed above that promote automatic thinking.

The *tachistoscope* exploits this threshold difference. It allows images or text to be shown for only brief periods of time. This time period can be adjusted so as to be above the threshold for subliminal perception, but below the threshold for conscious perception. This allows experimenters to expose subjects to purely unconscious stimuli and observe the effect they have on their behaviour.

Numerous experiments have been done using the tachistoscope that leave no doubt about the existence of the unconscious mind. What is more controversial is how, and in what ways, it differs from the conscious mind.

Experimental evidence for psychodynamic theory

Freud's psychodynamic theory is only based on case studies, but there is some experimental evidence to support certain aspects of it.

PERCEPTUAL DEFENCE

In *perceptual defence*, the unconscious mind withholds information from the conscious mind as if it is threatening. In an early experiment, participants were shown words that were either neutral, such as *apple*, or emotionally charged, such as *whore*. The length of time to which they were exposed to these words was slowly increased so that it passed from *below* the conscious threshold to *above* the conscious threshold. Participants were asked at which point they became aware of each word, and their skin conductivity was also monitored as a measure of their physiological stress. It was found that the emotionally charged words were recognised later than the neutral words, and that skin conductivity changes occurred before the reported recognition of the word.

SUBLIMINAL PSYCHODYNAMIC ACTIVATION

The theory of *subliminal psychodynamic activation* is that messages presented subliminally that contain elements of tension or stress (as opposed to reassurance or calm) can affect behaviour or cognitive performance without a person being aware of it. This effect has been demonstrated in a number of experiments. In one series, Silverman and colleagues tested Freud's theory that guilt over love for one's father is a source of stress that impairs performance in some females. Female undergraduate students were either shown the message *'Loving daddy is wrong'* or the message *'Loving daddy is okay'*. They were unaware of having been shown these messages, but after exposure they all underwent memory psychometric testing. The students performed poorly *only* if they had been exposed to *'Loving daddy is wrong'*.

Other experiments investigated the effect of the term *'Mamma is leaving me'* on the behaviour of people with eating disorders. The subjects were shown this phrase and similar phrases that were not emotionally loaded, such as *'Mamma is loaning it'*. Afterwards the subjects were given the opportunity to eat wheat crackers. They were all unaware of having been shown the phrases, but those with eating disorders who saw the phrase *'Mamma is leaving me'* ate significantly more crackers.

Current view of the unconscious

The unconscious is responsible for many – if not most – of our beliefs and actions. The current dominant view in psychology of the *cognitive unconscious* differs from that of Freud.

In this view, the unconscious does not have motivations that are hidden or independent of those of the conscious mind, and there is no special significance attached to biological motivations. Mental processes are unconscious because they do not receive the prominence necessary for them to cross the threshold into consciousness, or because they have become automatic by regular practice (as shown by activities like playing the piano, typing on a keyboard or tying shoelaces).

> According to this theory, the unconscious may provide *implicit motives* that we are not aware of – as opposed to *explicit motives* that we are aware of.

Implicit knowledge

Implicit learning and *implicit memory* refer to knowledge that we acquire and can then recall without any conscious awareness or the ability to verbalise. Examples are the grammatical rules we use when speaking in our mother tongue. Between the ages of 4 and 6, children have no notions of grammar but they still speak correctly because it *seems* right. There are two areas in which conscious and unconscious processing takes place in anatomically distinct locations.

- The first and most studied of these is in *vision*. There are extensive data on the difference between the conscious ventral visual stream to the visual cortex and the unconscious dorsal visual stream to the posterior parietal cortex.

- The second area is *memory*. Korsakoff's syndrome, head injury and strokes affect the fornices, mamillary bodies and medial temporal lobes of the brain. These conditions impair *explicit* memory, but leave implicit memory intact. The neurologist Claparède (1911) shook hands with a woman who was profoundly amnesic. In his hand he concealed a pin with which he pricked her. Afterward, she could not remember having her hand pricked, but she refused to shake hands with Claparède again. The reason she gave was that it was well known that people often hid pins in their hands.

Implicit memory or knowledge is:

- **Durable**—experiments in normal people show implicit knowledge is retained more reliably and for longer than explicit knowledge.

- **Holistic**—implicit knowledge is not linguistic but procedural in nature; it is also holistic, meaning that a sequence of letters like "P–Q" is not broken down into "P" and "Q" but remembered as a whole.

- **Inflexible**—subconscious knowledge requires stereotypical pattern recognition for its exercise; unlike conscious knowledge, it cannot be applied via analysis to unfamiliar situations.

- **Independent**—from explicit knowledge. Performance at implicit learning is consistent in any one person, so that people who do well on one experiment also tend to do well on others; however, there is little or no correlation with performance at explicit learning.

- **Has little age or IQ dependence**—this hypotheses is less well established but it seems implicit learning changes little with age or IQ, and shows lower variance in populations than explicit learning.

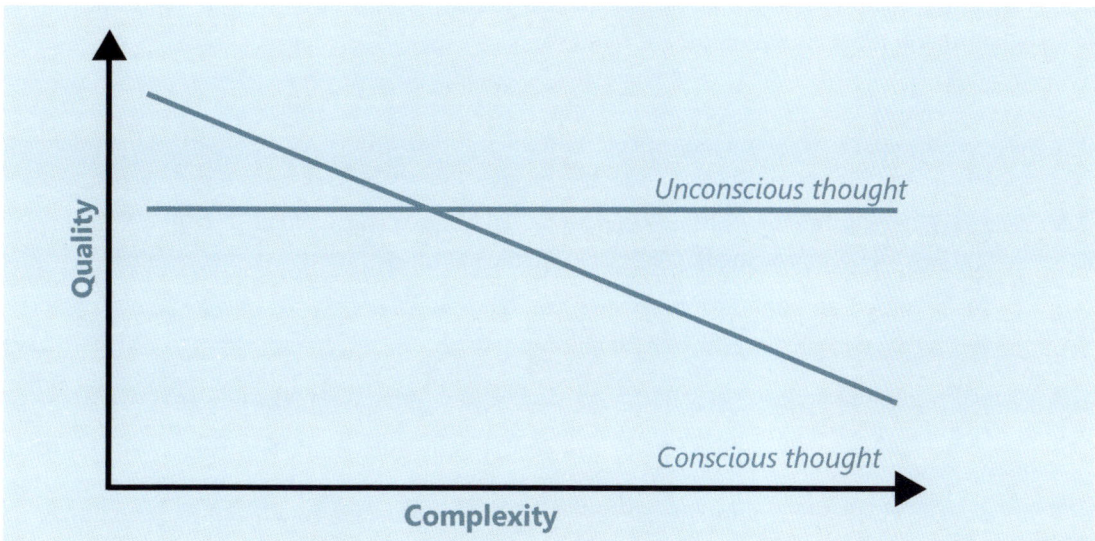

Figure 1.2 *The Unconscious Thought Theory (after Dijksterhuis and Nordgren, 2006).*

Unconscious decision-making

This topic is covered in *Module 2*. There are two theories about unconscious decision-making: the somatic marker hypothesis and the unconscious thought theory.

SOMATIC MARKER HYPOTHESIS

This suggests that unconscious cognitive processing leads to changes, such as 'gut feelings', which influence decision-making. Learning starts with an association between a perceived situation and an emotion. For example, you might be a cold dark room with blue light coming in through the window when something jumps out at you. This invokes fear and a 'fight or flight' response. When you are next in a cold dark room with a blue light, the fight or flight response may be invoked again and the somatic changes that occur may invoke fear.

UNCONSCIOUS THOUGHT THEORY

This concerns decision-making with information that is consciously accessible. The theory is that in highly complex situations and involved decisions, the quality of any decision is improved if the cognitive processing is subconscious (**Figure 1.2**). This kind of decision is taken by addressing an issue consciously, then 'sleeping on it' or turning attention elsewhere for a few days or weeks before returning to the question, if the solution does not 'pop into your head' first. The reverse is true of simple analytic decisions that are better taken directly in consciousness.

Emotion

A lot has been learned about emotions and the brain regions that control them from brain-damaged patients, such as the now well-known rail-road worker Phineas Gage who suffered a penetrating brain injury in 1848. He recovered but lost all emotional feelings and he was unable to plan or structure his life. More recent studies have made similar findings. Such brain-damaged people have defects in the late stages of reasoning; their weighting and selection of options is random and occurs without planning. Normal social functioning is not possible for them.

- The emotions form the communication pathway from the unconscious mind to the conscious mind and are responsible for all human motivation.
- Emotion drives the affect heuristic, in which emotional "tags" (positive or negative) are generated by a situation, and promote a rapid judgement or decision.
- Specific emotions have specific features. For example, anger promotes automatic thinking and also leads people to blame other individuals, rather than the situation, for bad things. It is reduced by changing to analytic thinking.
- Positive emotions give durable increases in physical, social and intellectual resources for coping with stress. People experiencing positive emotions are more capable of "stepping back" from their current problems and to "consider them from multiple angles".

The interaction between emotion and cognition is not always beneficial and any inappropriate or high level of emotion can interfere with attention, memory and logical reasoning. The consequences may be a loss of flexibility in thinking and an inability to consider alternatives, as well as causing distraction, poor concentration and a distorted world view.

Chronic stress can cause significant somatic health problems. It can lead to:

- Cell death in the hippocampal region of the brain, which causes memory loss.
- Clinical depression and anxiety states.

Admiral Kimmel was the Commander of the American Fleet in Pearl Harbour during the air attack of 1941. Despite increasing intelligence reports of an impending raid, he failed to take measures to defend his base and his fleet was destroyed as a consequence. It has been suggested that this happened because rational decision making was impaired by stress and fear.

Similar processes may have been involved in the response to the 1918–1919 influenza pandemic. Despite rising rates of infection and increasing numbers of deaths, there was widespread prevarication and denial amongst most public health departments and, with few exceptions, it was fatal inertia that lead to the large-scale mortality that ensued.

Decision Making

Key points for reflection

1. Understand the difference between automatic and analytic decision-making.

2. Learning progresses from conscious incompetence to unconscious competence via conscious competence. We are at different points on this pathway for different areas of knowledge or experience.

We divide decisions into automatic versus analytic and conscious versus unconscious. When choosing a new car we decide in analytic mode. We read brochures, try out different models and discuss colours and the deals available, the select the option we like best. When driving the car many decisions are automatic. We stop at red lights, we decide to go the correct way on familiar routes.

Analytic decision making

Analytic decisions are those for which we have the time and information to consider various options and gain further information as necessary. Early research was done on this type of decision and led to the classical theory of the specific steps we go through in making a decision:

- Step 0—Decision trigger
- Step 1—Assessment
- Step 2—Options checking
- Step 3—Project and decide
- Step 4—Review

Step 0: Decision trigger

The decision trigger is not actually part of decision-making, and that is why it is numbered as 0. It is part of situation awareness (SA) and is covered in detail in the triggered check SA model in Module 3.

Step 1: Assessment

This involves assessing the consequences of the decision and the time and resources available to make it, rather than the decision itself. This involves questions like:

- What is the ultimate objective?
- How long have I got?
- Do I have all the facts?
- What are the risks?

However, the ultimate objective is often overlooked! Is it:

- Treating more people or curing more disease?
- Prolonging life or reducing suffering?
- Reducing costs or increasing profits?
- Disciplining a staff member or improving patient safety?

Getting the ultimate objective right leads to new (and often better) options.

Inexperienced decision-makers tend to hurry to the first available option. Time is rarely as pressured as that so it is usually better to prolong the mental assessment process at the expense of reduced time for action.

Consider making a decision to operate for appendicitis. Relevant features to look out for in the patient include a coated tongue, rebound peritonism, anorexia, and tender groin lymph nodes. Less relevant features are the patient's hair colour, tendon reflexes and visual acuity. The surgeon gathers the relevant information by specifically looking for it. This is true generally. The best assessments identify the most important factors out of a large number of features, which are specifically looked for.

Step 2: Options checking

The options checking idea was developed for this course. It is a mental habit analogous to the situation awareness (SA) check discussed in *Module 3*. It is a practical, take-home message.

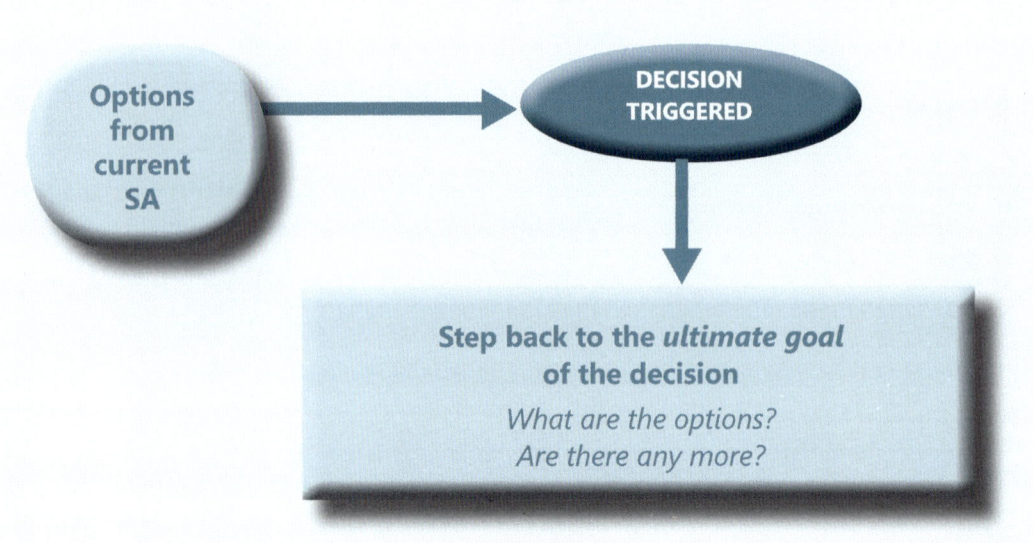

Figure 2.1 *The options check.*

The check begins with the conscious identification of the ultimate objective of the decision, as well as the options in hand. Then it involves stepping back to see if there are further options that have not yet been considered.

Options checking has been described as creative or adaptive decision-making. Decisions with particularly thorough and creative options checking make good stories and can lead to new practices or ways of thinking. Option checking is at its best when *no existing options look attractive.*

> **Vignette 2.1 Option checking at 35,000 feet**
>
> Orthopaedic surgeon, Professor Wallace, was travelling from Hong Kong to London when he was asked to care for a passenger who had developed chest pain after being involved in a motorcycle accident before boarding the plane. The passenger rapidly became unwell.
>
> The professor suspected a pneumothorax, which happens when a damaged lung leaks air that becomes trapped and threatens life. With minimal aids to diagnosis, he asked for a second opinion from Doctor Wong, who was also on the plane. Doctor Wong agreed with the diagnosis.
>
> They then improvised a chest drain set. They used a urinary catheter, a coat-hanger as a trocar, sellotape, oxygen tubing and a plastic bottle of mineral water as a water trap. They used five-star brandy as a disinfectant. The patient recovered.

The doctors initially had no attractive options for treating the passenger. They asked for advice from the ground about what equipment was on board – but none came. They considered a flight diversion, but time was too short. The catheter in the aircraft's medical kit would work as a drain, but it would let air into the chest as well as letting it out. Therefore they needed a one-way valve system, so they devised one from whatever was at hand. Their option checking was prompted because initially there was no attractive option. This is often the case, and is precisely why "necessity is the mother of invention".

> **Vignette 2.2 Option checking for airway control**
>
> A patient (now referred to as Chuck!) used an electric drill in a suicide attempt. He damaged one of his carotid arteries and his trachea. When he got to A&E the drill bit was still there, passing into his damaged trachea, which was partially obstructed and bleeding. As the drill bit was removed, a wire was introduced into the trachea through the entry wound, enabling dilation and then intubation, and airway control.

The standard options for emergency airway control are intubation via the mouth, and surgical tracheostomy. In this case, neither option was attractive. The drill bit was passing through the trachea, and blood and swelling were obscuring the surgical and laryngoscopic (intubation) views. Simply removing the drill risked closing the airway and there would be insufficient time to re-open it. By placing a guidewire through the wound into the trachea, they were able to remove the drill bit and confidently place an endotracheal tube in the right place quickly.

Step 3: Project and decide

Projecting an option means predicting its consequences (or its *utility*). In this step, each option is projected and the option with the best consequences is chosen. The projecting options in **Vignette 2.2** went like this:

> **Option 1**—*Orally intubate the patient in the conventional fashion*
> This was tried, but it failed.
>
> **Option 2**—*Create a surgical airway*
> This was considered, but projection indicated that there was a high risk that the damaged trachea would be difficult to identify and cannulate from a conventional tracheostomy incision, and there could be a long delay between removing the drill bit and securing the airway. This delay might lead to critical hypoxia. On the basis of this projection, Option 2 was rejected.
>
> **Option 3**—*Intubate via the wound*
> The possibility of intubation via the wound seemed feasible using a guidewire technique. Projection indicated uncertainty about the feasibility of passing the guidewire, but if it failed nothing was lost. If it succeeded, however, it projected a high probability of removal of the drill followed by rapid and accurate intubation. The decision was made and the projection proved correct.

ACCURACY VERSUS UTILITY OF PROJECTIONS

Accuracy versus utility is a mathematical model of decision-making. Suppose again you have to decide whether or not to remove a patient's appendix. If you choose to go ahead and the appendix turns out to be normal, that option would have been incorrect. If you choose not to perform the operation, and the patient makes a rapid and full recovery, then the no surgery option was the correct one. We define an option's accuracy as the probability that it will prove correct.

An option's utility relates to its consequences, whether or not it is correct. With the appendectomy decision, the utility of the option to operate has the positive component of potential cure if it is correct. And it has the negative component of an unnecessary operation if it is not.

> **Mathematical calculation of utility**
>
> $$\begin{pmatrix} \text{Probability that the option} \\ \text{is correct (accuracy)} \end{pmatrix} \times \begin{pmatrix} \text{A measure of its consequences} \\ \text{if correct} \end{pmatrix}$$
>
> $$+$$
>
> $$\begin{pmatrix} \text{Probability that the option} \\ \text{is incorrect (1 − accuracy)} \end{pmatrix} \times \begin{pmatrix} \text{A measure of its consequences} \\ \text{if incorrect} \end{pmatrix}$$

Module Two: Decision Making

Ultimately it is *utility* rather than *accuracy* that drives decision-making.

In the case of **Vignette 2.3** the accuracy of the option to place a guidewire through the wound (i.e. the chance of success) was not known and perhaps not thought to be high, but the utility was high. The consequence of success was quick and safe intubation; the consequence of failing to get the wire in the right place was no harm done!

> Here is an extreme example. You are going sailing. Should you wear a life-jacket? If you decide to wear one, it will be the correct option if you fall in the water and cannot swim to safety. This is highly improbable, however, so the accuracy of the option is very low. Utility shows that the cost of this option – if incorrect – is low. You just have to wear a not uncomfortable jacket. The utility if the option is correct will save your life! Ergo you wear it.

Both accuracy and utility can be improved by identifying and gathering relevant information, and this improves what is called decision quality. For a given decision quality, there is a trade-off between accuracy and utility. The mathematical model is used to optimise this trade-off when deciding things like the best diagnostic criteria for cancer screening programs.

Step 4: Review

In the review stage, the decision is re-visited in the light of updated information. This information is used for two purposes:

- To suggest new options (a positive options check is an important part of review).
- To update projections of the option – the one that was chosen and the others.

Weaknesses of analytic decision making

Vignette 2.5 shows a weakness of analytic decision-making.

> ### Vignette 2.3   Too little glucose
>
> A 32-year-old woman with kidney failure was admitted with internal bleeding that needed surgery. She had a dangerously high potassium level of 8.5 mmol/L. The A&E consultant prescribed insulin to lower her potassium and a glucose drip to counter the reduction in glucose that insulin causes.
>
> Five minutes into the operation, the anaesthetist requested blood for a transfusion. She had been told blood was being cross-matched and was therefore surprised that the lab had no record! Rapidly organising sampling and cross-matching, she gave the patient fluid for volume replacement, and two units of O-negative blood. She was delighted to achieve stability until the cross-matched blood arrived fifty minutes later.
>
> After the operation the patient did not wake up. The anaesthetist did a blood sugar test and was horrified to find that it was dangerously low, less than 0.5 mmol/L. The patient had sustained irreversible brain damage from which she died ten days later. The glucose and insulin regimen had become a distant memory, displaced by other immediate pressures.

The anaesthetist's single analytic channel was committed to the problem of replacing blood loss and this blocked it to all other issues. The more relaxed, regular situation awareness checks that she would have performed were missed, which is why she missed the glucose issue.

If during the briefing she had made a mental note like 'Chemical state: potassium, insulin, glucose – risks!' her automatic mind would have been primed.

Experimental evidence shows that automatic thinking can be primed. People notice things they are told to look out for, even if they do not remember being told. Warning inexperienced staff of potential risks to be aware of is worth it, even if they do not appear to take the information on board!

Advantages and disadvantages of analytic thinking are listed below.

Table 2.1 *Advantages and disadvantages of analytic decisions*

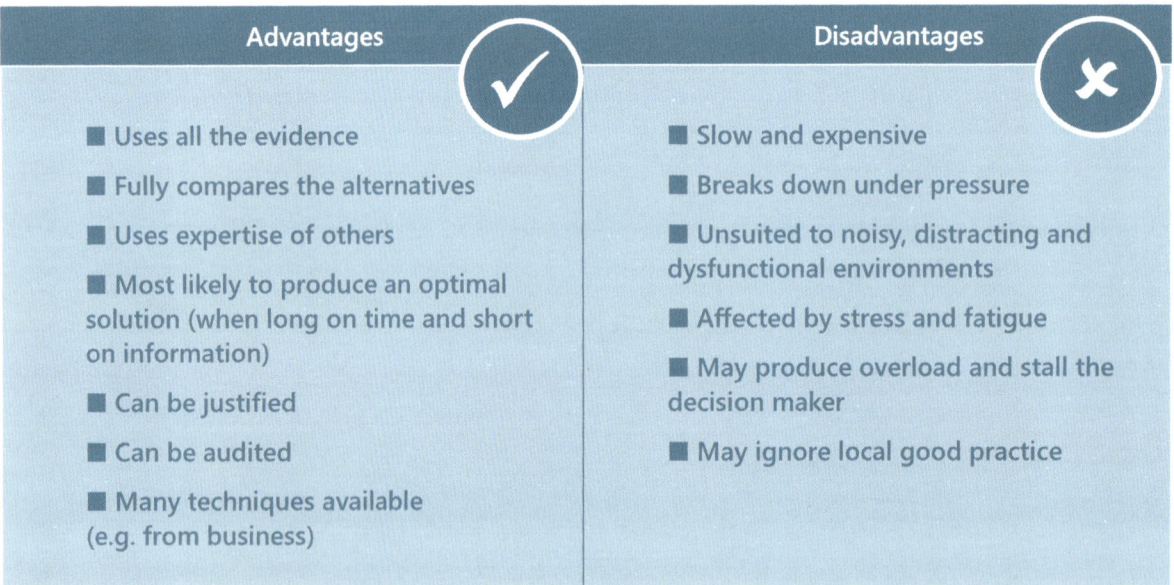

Advantages ✓	Disadvantages ✗
■ Uses all the evidence	■ Slow and expensive
■ Fully compares the alternatives	■ Breaks down under pressure
■ Uses expertise of others	■ Unsuited to noisy, distracting and dysfunctional environments
■ Most likely to produce an optimal solution (when long on time and short on information)	■ Affected by stress and fatigue
■ Can be justified	■ May produce overload and stall the decision maker
■ Can be audited	■ May ignore local good practice
■ Many techniques available (e.g. from business)	

Rule-based decisions

Rule-based decisions are made by consciously applying a rule which is usually imposed from outside, rather than derived by the individual. These decisions involve fitting the situation to the appropriate rule; lack of situational flexibility is their problem.

Vignette 2.4 Fire at Turkey Creek Bridge

A Union Pacific coal train of 100 trucks was travelling from Denver to Chicago when an axle-bearing on the 57th truck failed and overheated. The crew noticed smoke and sparks and so they stopped the train. The faulty truck, however, was about half a mile behind the engine, so by the time they reached it the wooden bridge the train had stopped on was on fire.

They uncoupled as many trucks as they could from the burning section, leaving six to fall into the creek as the bridge burned. No-one was hurt, but the total losses were estimated at over $2,000,000 ($250,000 for the trucks and over $1,750,000 for the bridge).

Union Pacific had a rule for this situation, which was to stop the train immediately a bearing failed. It was a sensible rule, but following it to the letter with a white-hot bearing over a timber-constructed bridge that had been recently creosoted was not a good decision.

Here is another example. Anticoagulants are given after operations to prevent deep venous thrombosis that can lead to a lethal pulmonary embolus. Dealing with this is usually a rule-based decision. A rule that all post-operative patients must receive an anticoagulant means it may be given inappropriately to people who are allergic to them, or who are prone to bleeding (such as those with stomach ulcers).

Both examples – the axle-bearing and the post-op anticoagulants – can be accommodated in rule-based decisions by including exceptions into more complex protocols. However, the rules then become cumbersome, slow to apply, and difficult to remember.

A risky rule-based decision is involved when applying high-minded platitudes. Phrases like *Safety first*, *Honesty is the best policy* and *The patient comes first* do not represent universal truths, but frequent opinions in straightforward situations.

Difficult analytical decisions are hard to make and it is tempting to reach for a platitude as a shortcut to an answer. The situations to which they are directly applicable are generally easy to resolve. If a decision is hard, then platitudes are probably not appropriate!

Table 2.2 *Advantages and disadvantages of rule-based decisions*

Advantages ✓	Disadvantages ✗
■ Good for novices	■ May not suit new situations
■ No need to understand reasoning behind each step	■ There is not a rule for every situation
■ Rapid, (if the rule is known)	■ A rule that does exist may not be known or not be found
■ Course of action has expert backing	■ If interrupted, may miss a vital step
■ Uses available evidence of good practice	■ May not understand reasoning, leading to risk of wrong procedure being selected
■ Produces consistency	■ Can produce unthinking compliance
■ Easy to justify	■ May stifle creativity
■ Allows managerial control and audit	■ Can be time-consuming (if rule not known)
■ Many good decisions come from following rules	

Rule-based decisions should not be seen as a separate category of decision, but as providing options for analytical decision-making.

When presented with a rule-based decision, consider the steps of assessment, options checking (applying the rule is one option), project and decide, and review.

Automatic decisions

Automatic decisions are also called recognition-primed, pattern recognition or intuitive decisions. We recognise a situation, refer to our prior knowledge of it, and use that knowledge to decide what to do. With familiarity, such decisions become both automatic and unconscious. When we drive to work, we may be completely preoccupied with matters that are unrelated to navigation, yet at each road junction we still "decide" to go the correct way.

When researchers studied real-life decisions made by experienced people they found that earlier analytic models from laboratory experiments did not fit. This lead to the use of the terms *classical* decision theory, for the experimental analytic type, and *naturalistic* decision theory, for the real-life automatic type.

Automatic decisions are our default way of managing everyday activities. These include things like dressing, breakfasting and driving. They are fast and involve low effort and they usually work well, however they are prone to matching the wrong pattern.

> **Vignette 2.5 Misleading asthma severity**
>
> A junior A&E doctor was treating a man with an asthma attack. The man had had several recent admissions with severe attacks and this time was unable to speak. Chest examination found there was little wheezing, and this comforted the doctor. He then tried, with some difficulty, to get the rest of the history.
>
> The patient's consciousness level suddenly deteriorated and the heart monitor showed cardiac arrest was imminent! After a few minutes of activity, the patient was safely anaesthetised and ventilated, and receiving treatment for severe asthma and a precipitating chest infection.

This doctor used faulty automatic decision-making and failed to change to analytic mode. He matched a simplistic pattern (asthma makes people wheeze: more wheeze = worse asthma; less wheeze = less severe asthma) and the patient's relatively quiet chest made him match it to the mild attack pattern. Therefore, he managed it accordingly. He could not pattern match correctly because he had no prior experience of this type of case, but he had been told about it during his training. If he had changed to analytic mode and assessed the situation with other guides to severity of the attack (such as measurement of peak airflow or blood gases), he would have got it right.

> If someone lacks experience, analytic decision-making can compensate, but it has to be engaged.

Experienced doctors rapidly narrow a diagnosis down to two or three likely possibilities and ask specific questions that distinguish between them. This rapid and effective system depends on much automatic-decision making and a little analytic. A far longer list of diagnostic options is taught to students for any given conditions. The contrast is because teaching can only inform an analytic approach, while the automatic approach requires experience.

> ### Vignette 2.6 Ruptured heart valve
>
> A cardiologist came to the assistance of a young doctor whose heart patient had suddenly become very sick. Within seconds he recognised the distinctive murmur of a ruptured heart string. Immediate open heart surgery saved the patient following his rapid and accurate decision. In this scenario, the cardiologist was unaware of any thought processes in coming to his decision.

> ### Vignette 2.7 The Gimli glider
>
> In 1983, a Boeing 767 ran out of fuel at 41,000 feet because of a ground crew error. The plane's engines failed. The flight manual contained no instructions for this particular situation. The nearest airfield was Gimli, a former Canadian Air Force base that had only a short runway. On approach, the powerless Boeing was too high, but aiming lower would make the aircraft gain speed and over-run the airway. The crew considered performing a full 360-degree turn in order to lose height, but they projected that they would lose too much.
>
> The Captain had past gliding experience. One gliding technique used in this situation is known as a "slide-slip" whereby the glider is flown slightly side-on to the wind to increase the drag and therefore lose height without gaining speed. This is not taught to commercial pilots, and it was not in the manual.
>
> The pilot successfully side-slipped and landed accurately. The plane was damaged but later repaired, but not one of the sixty-one passengers or crew were injured. When the manoeuvre was later tried on a simulator it failed to model the behaviour of the Boeing accurately.

The decision to use side-slipping was an analytic one with decisive options checking! Once decided, the actions were taken automatically from the Captain's previous experience.

The danger of pattern matching is in picking the wrong pattern. Then, unless the pattern is corrected to the right one – or changed to analytic decision-making – a poor decision will be made. Increasing experience makes us better at recognising more patterns and so increases our ability to use this method. At the same time, however, it reduces our tendency to use analytic decision making.

Rule-based automatic decisions

Rule-based decisions become automatic when we are practised at them. One example is stopping at a red traffic light. These decisions are specific to their context and are resistant to change if the context changes. Driving in other countries with alternative traffic signals is an example of this. Original learning interferes with new learning, and the more experienced you are with one system, the more interference there will be with the new learning.

Not all automatic decisions are good decisions (such as, deciding to smoke another cigarette) and they can be particularly difficult when policy changes are planned. Concern about hospital-acquired infections in the UK prompted policy changes on dress and hand-washing by ward staff. Automatic learning (habits) interfered with this policy change. After considerable exposure, discussion and effort, however, the new policy did become an automatic rule-based behaviour.

Table 2.3 *Advantages and disadvantages of automatic decisions*

Advantages ✓	Disadvantages ✗
■ Very fast	■ Requires experience
■ Robust (most of the time)	■ Often is (or becomes) unconscious
■ Useful in routine situations	■ Does not deal well with the unfamiliar
■ Little conscious thought required	■ May not prompt a situation awareness check when things change or should be reviewed
■ Overloaded less easily than other modes	■ Hard to explain or justify later
	■ Prone to the limitations of heuristics

Unconscious decision-making

In automatic decision-making there is a role for unconscious processing that leads to something appearing in consciousness without apparently having been considered. This depends on implicit knowledge that is learned incidentally to what we are doing without our knowing it. This type of learning does not depend on attention or working memory.

Two theories in psychology address unconscious decision-making:

- the somatic marker hypothesis
- the unconscious thought theory.

Somatic marker hypothesis

The somatic marker hypothesis is that unconscious cognitive processing leads to conscious correlates such as "gut feelings". These influence decision making, as well as certain physiological changes, such as the "cold sweat" of fear.

The response is controlled by a specific brain area, as shown in patients who have suffered damage to this area; they have normal intellectual cognitive performance, but profoundly disrupted social behaviour, which often leads them to disastrous decision-making.

Examples of the somatic marker effects include the uneasy feeling of impending trouble. An experienced fire-chief called all his troops out of a burning building just seconds before it collapsed. When asked to explain why, he said he did not know and denied even making a decision. He just did it. In this case, an automatic decision was influenced by an unconscious marker based on previous experience of burning buildings that collapsed.

Such decisions can be hard to explain to observers and hard to justify to superiors when they pay off badly. They are possibly hard to justify even when they go well, since they may appear to divert from the rules and therefore subvert their main purpose (in this case, stopping the building from burning down).

Unconscious thought theory

Unconscious thought theory is like 'sleeping on' a problem. It holds that the analytical solution of problems can be made in the conscious or the unconscious mind. In the latter case, the solution starts with conscious consideration of the problem. Conscious attention is then transferred elsewhere while the unconscious analysis continues. The solution then re-emerges into consciousness, usually at times of relaxation.

This phenomenon has led to the "Three Bs" of creative innovation – the Bus the Bath and the Bed. The unconscious thought theory holds that in highly complex situations and involved decisions, the quality of decisions is improved if the cognitive processing is unconscious. The reverse is true of simple decisions (**Figure 2.2**).

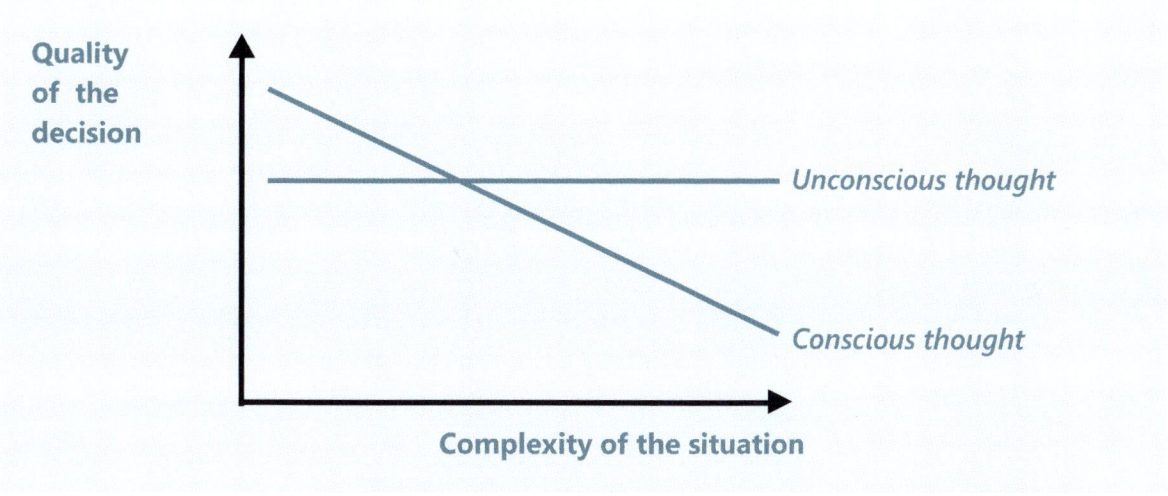

Figure 2.2 *Graph of unconscious thought theory, showing the effect of quality and complexity of a situation on thought.*

Group decisions

Groups can develop and sustain good or poor decision-making practice. In a study of teams using X-ray screening to detect cracks in aircraft wings, there were some effective teams and some less effective teams. New members joining one of the high-performing teams gravitated to a high level of performance. In the poorer teams, the new members gravitated towards poorer performance levels. Some of those who performed well in effective teams also performed poorly in the poor-performing teams.

Group decisions require conscious communication by group members and this requires that such decisions are analytic, and have the same components as individual analytical decisions: that is:

- **Step 1**—Assessment
- **Step 2**—Options checking
- **Step 3**—Project and decide
- **Step 4**—Review

Step 1—Assessment

It is particularly important in groups to be clear about the decision's ultimate objective.

Step 2—Options checking

People who are aware of pertinent information should express that knowledge, if it is not already in discussion. This can be difficult for people who are introverted. Conversely, other members of a group should not impede the input of others by being unduly overbearing or dismissive. In groups, suggesting imaginative and favourable options can attract credit as well as hostility from those who feel under threat. Group leaders have a duty to identify such options when suggested, to use credit appropriately and to distinguish between the issue and the people.

Step 3—Project and decide

In multidisciplinary teams, different specialists can accurately project different options: surgeons for operations, physicians for drugs, and so on. With good projections, choosing the option with the highest utility is usually straightforward. In groups, the skill in choosing lies in assessing the quality and accuracy of the projections, particularly the projections of creative suggestions that may have great advantages but which the group's members may have little experience of. The role of the group leader is not generally to take the decision, but rather to elicit the best quality options and projections until one winner is clear. If the leader makes the decision prematurely they are likely to alienate other group members as well as make a bad decision.

Step 4—Review

Review is often not carried out by the group that made the decision. After a group decision has been made about patient treatment, individual clinicians only are present when further information becomes available, from which projections can be updated and new options considered. It may not be feasible to take the new information back to the original group, but the same decision-making processes is followed.

Conclusions

Decision theory, cognitive processing, and situation awareness are all intimately linked to each other. Many of the aspects covered in this **module** overlap with parallel aspects of the other **modules**, and it is suggested that topics such as the triggered situation awareness check, analytic thinking, automatic thinking and unconscious processing are revised together.

Situation Awareness

Key points for reflection

❶ We often do not see or misinterpret evidence that does not support our initial hypotheses. It is important actively to note such evidence as part of a continuous process of situation assessment.

❷ You cannot stop fixation happening but be aware of it in others and its potential in yourself.

Situation awareness (SA) is our mental picture of what is happening around us and of what is about to happen. SA is important because of how easily it can become dangerously faulty. There are plenty of examples of this. The Silva *USS Montana* advertisement can be seen on the e-learning part of this course (www.safercare.eu/human/) or on *You Tube*.

Vignette 3.1 The lost car

After work one evening, you go to the car park as normal but you cannot find your car – a tall people-carrier with a roof-box on the top (very easy to spot). You search the car park in vain and finally consider other options for getting home (and informing the police that it has been stolen). However, the reason you cannot find it is because you have driven to work in your *partner's* car.

Being an experienced driver does not prevent SA problems like this. In this scenario, you are not distracted; you are concentrating on the issue. A lack of driving experience would not stop a child from solving the problem.

The wrong diagnosis is a common SA error in medicine.

The scenario described in **Vignette 3.2** happened in the 1990s when more X-ray examinations than endoscopies were used to investigate bowel disease.

> ### Vignette 3.2 Crohn's or appendicitis
>
> A boy aged 8 presented with abdominal pain and diarrhoea. The house-officer found non-specific tenderness and mild fever, and wrote "Possible appendicitis but not typical. Inflammatory bowel disease? Enteritis?"
>
> The paediatricians arranged a barium enema. This showed an area of irregularity in the large bowel consistent with Crohn's disease. In a clinical meeting, the radiologist deemed the diagnosis "uncertain". A trial of treatment was commenced with the intention of reviewing the diagnosis in the light of the boy's response. The drugs used for Crohn's disease suppress the body's defence against infection. The boy seemed to improve for two days, then he relapsed. A second drug was added and his condition stabilised over the next few days. Again he deteriorated.
>
> His case was discussed again. The original plan had been forgotten about and discussion now focused on how to manage his refractory (i.e. not responding to treatment) Crohn's disease. The treatment was changed again. This went on for three weeks.
>
> Surgical resection of the bowel is an option for Crohn's disease but it does not cure the disease, and it leads to loss of bowel and possibly the need for a colostomy, but there seemed to be no alternative. The surgeon did not find Crohn's disease but appendicitis! After three weeks on immunosuppressive treatment and no antibiotics the infection was rampant – the worst case the surgeon had seen. The boy made a full recovery.

Cases like this start with a tentative assessment. The focus then shifts onto dealing with the situation as perceived, without returning to the assessment. If that assessment is incorrect, things go wrong. Notice these features:

- The problem is a mistaken mental model of the situation – the wrong diagnosis.
- It arose because critical information was presented in an error-prone manner.
- Before the operation, the boy was sick but the doctors were calm. There was no hint that they were part of the problem.
- During this time the problem would have been easy to correct if it had been recognised.
- The way to fix the problem was to return to the assessment stage and do an "SA check".

> ### Vignette 3.3 Wrong-side eye surgery
>
> Malignant melanoma is a cancer that can arise in the eye. It causes blindness in the eye and becomes fatal if it is not controlled. Treatment is the surgical removal of the eyeball. This operation was planned on a man with a melanoma in his left eye. He was marked for the operation.
>
> In theatre, the first drape inadvertently covered the mark above his left eye. When the scrub nurse went to pick up the second drape, the stack of drapes fell to the floor. There was a short delay while new drapes were opened, then draping continued – but around the right eye.

Everything seemed calm and normal, but the team was heading for a disaster. Notice the parallels with the case above:

- The problem is a mistaken mental model – this time, that the surgeons were proceeding with the correct eye.
- It arose because the circumstances made the presentation of crucial information error prone.
- All remained calm in theatre.
- The problem could be easily corrected if it were recognised in time.

The hospital had previously introduced a strict checking system before any scrub nurse even handed a scalpel to a surgeon. In this way, the error was spotted. The patient was re-draped and the operation was performed on the correct eye.

Triggered checks

Accurate SA is maintained using so-called triggered checks. These have two components:

- The SA check.
- The things that trigger it.

The SA check

There are three stages in the SA check process.

- First—identify the features of the current SA, then step back to consider other possible hypotheses.
- Second—consider and (ideally) verbalise all the alternative hypotheses.
- Third—seek external evidence to decide between the alternatives.

The point to step back to is the last one, when the SA was correct – but when was this? The most recent point that passes the SA check is of no help if the SA was faulty before then! You should question whether, for the task in hand, the SA could always have been wrong. If the SA started correct, it presumably has not changed, but the situation may have. You should work sequentially through past events, doing the same check for each point until reaching the present. This sounds more difficult than it is in reality. As with all checks that fail, in most cases it is not because they were not done correctly, but because they were not done at all. Examples of SA checks based on the vignettes are given below.

TRIGGERS FOR SA CHECKS

SA checks are triggered by checking schedules or things we notice. Reliable SA depends on having a low threshold for triggering checks.

TRIGGERS THAT ARE NOTICED

These are events that can attract our attention. The more familiar we are with how things should be, the more sensitive we become to things that are not expected. However, whatever our level of experience, there are other factors that also determine whether we notice clues. The more engaged we are with a task, for example, the less we notice other things and the more obvious they have to be before we do notice them.

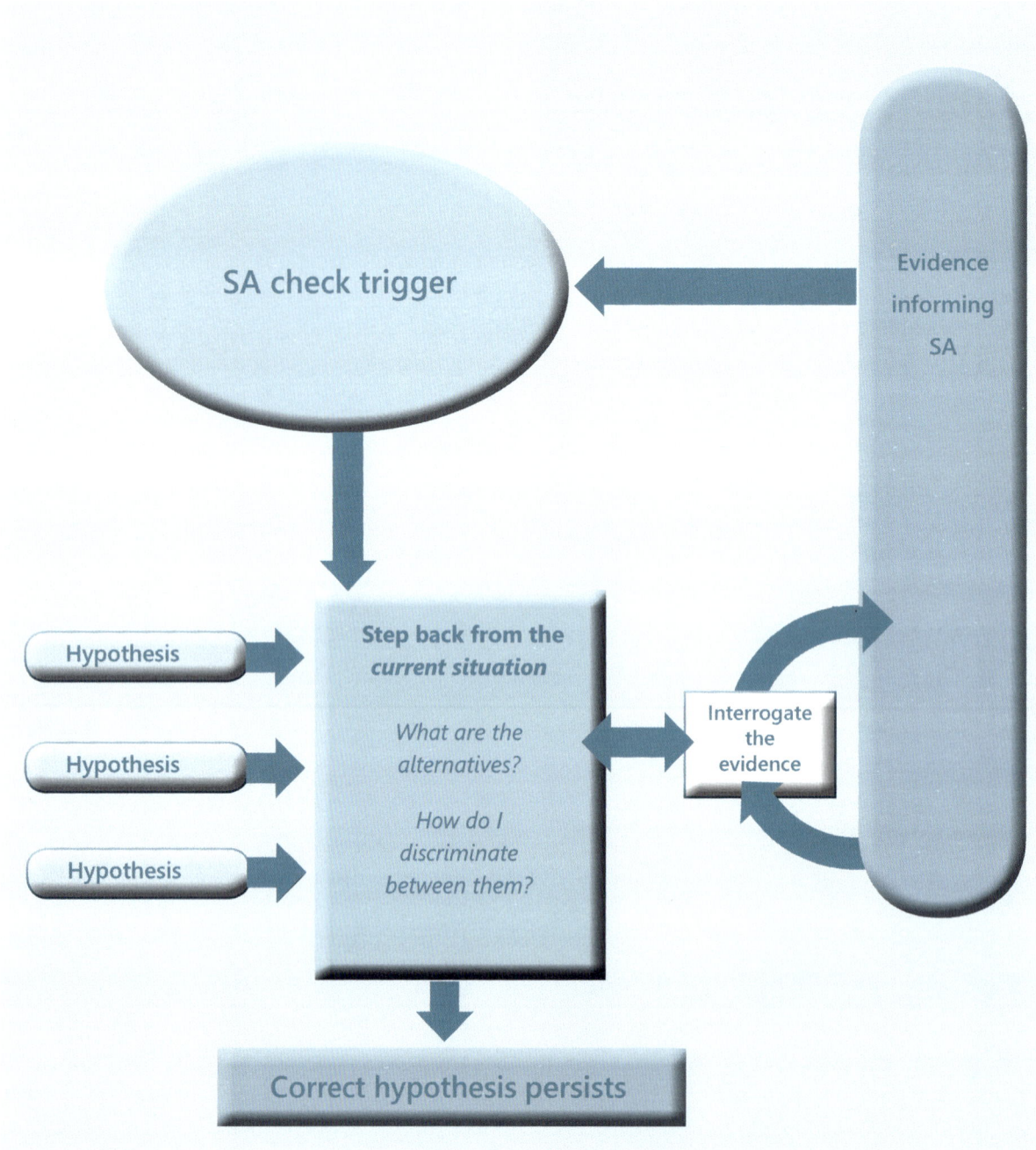

Figure 3.1 *The situation awareness (SA) check.*

In the extreme this is called fixation, where one issue so engrosses us that we become unaware of an obvious change in the situation that is more significant than what we are concentrating on. Consider these examples of fixation:

- Fixation on intubation (while hypoxia develops that should prompt a surgical airway).
- Fixation on repairing a bleeding vein (while a patient exsanguinates) that should be packed pending haemodynamic stabilisation.
- Fixation on gaining intravenous access (when the situation demands administration of drugs via any route).

Film clips are available that engage the viewer's attention while slipping something "obvious" past so that the viewer misses it. Examples are a series of short films by Transport for London that aim to promote awareness of cyclists among drivers. They work because fixation is made less likely by knowing about it.

Other things that make us liable to miss clues are:

- Fatigue.
- Stress.
- Negative emotional states.

TRIGGERS THAT ARE NOT NOTICED

These are clues that are not events and do not attract our attention. They can be steady or slowly changing features and changes in inconspicuous instruments. Or they can be things that should be there but are not, or things that should not be there but are, or things in the wrong place. Spotting these clues can be helped by checklists and by turning features into events. Many monitored parameters, such as blood oxygen levels, are turned into events by the use of warning bleeps or lights.

SA checks take a degree of cognitive effort and we avoid them by dismissing triggers. We naturally resist changing out mental models. When new facts arrive that challenge our model, our instinct is to rationalise the facts to fit the model, rather than change the model to fit the facts. If a clue fits our model, we are more likely to notice it, interpret it correctly and consider it to be important than if it does not.

This is called confirmation bias. When clues are open to more than one interpretation, we pick the one that fits our current model, rather than looking for alternative models and deciding which model the clues fit best.

Vignette 3.4 Tumour-related brain swelling

A young woman had an operation to remove a brain tumour. The surgeons had planned to remove it through the space between the two sides of the brain, However, when they began to do so, they found the swelling became too severe to proceed. There are several causes of intra-operative brain swelling, only one of which is a tumour. In this case, swelling had not been expected because the tumour was small; nonetheless the surgeons thought it the likeliest cause. They changed the operative approach, but the swelling still impeded their progress. Some cerebrospinal fluid was drained which reduced the swelling so that the tumour could be successfully removed.

Tumour-related swelling should recede when a tumour is removed, but in this case it got even worse until it became life-threatening. An ultrasound scan was used to look for a haemorrhage in the tumour bed that might be causing it, but none was seen. The range of the scanner was increased from a few centimetres, the range for the tumour bed, to a greater range so that the whole brain could be seen. Something was seen that should not have been there – a blood clot pressing on the opposite side of the brain.

They realised the swelling had been due to this clot developing on the other side. The operative wound was hastily closed and a craniotomy performed on the other side. An extensive extradural clot was removed. The swelling disappeared and the patient's pulse and blood pressure returned to normal. She made a full recovery.

The surgeons' mental model was that the swelling was caused by the tumour. As time passed, clues appeared that were less and less consistent with this model, but they were interpreted as confirming it, and the SA became dangerously wrong. Evidence then emerged that did not fit the SA and it was corrected in time.

The SA trigger list

Investigations of accidents from many walks of life have found that SA-related adverse events are often preceded by one or more of these stereotypical patterns, and by enough time that the adverse events could have been avoided if the pattern had triggered an SA check.

AN ACTION DOES NOT HAVE THE EXPECTED EFFECT

A clue to the wrong diagnosis is that the patient does not respond as expected to treatment.

CONFUSION OR UNCERTAINTY NOT RESOLVED

Uncertainty is common with junior staff or staff seeking clarity on issues outside their specialist field. The habit of doing an SA check if you are uncertain is clearly valuable, but there is another message: when you are in a senior position with others looking up to you for clarification, do an SA check whenever you detect uncertainty in them. This habit alone would have prevented countless disasters (like the one in **Vignette 3.8**).

DISAGREEMENT BETWEEN TWO SOURCES OF INFORMATION

Two conflicting sources of information cannot both be right. Work out which is which from other evidence – do not just pick the one that fits your current mental model.

FIXATION ON A SINGLE TASK

This is hard to spot in oneself, but easier to see in others, for example if they are not responding to questions. If someone else thinks you are fixating, they are probably right.

LEADING QUESTIONS

Leading questions seek confirmation of one interpretation of the situation, rather than looking for others. Asking "The blood pressure is stable, isn't it?" is a leading question, but "Is the blood pressure stable?" is not.

DISPLACEMENT ACTIVITIES

These are behaviour patterns that seem out of context with the situation, or with the behaviour that occurs immediately before or after them. They occur when people are in situations they cannot control or cope with. Typical displacement activities are scratching of the head, humming a tune, doodling on paper, or fiddling with small objects.

FAILURE TO ADHERE TO ACCEPTED PRACTICE

If a team member is deviating from standard practice it may be because they are not aware what the standard practice is, or they may have reason to believe that the standard practice is sub-optimal; or it might be because either they or you have standard practice for the wrong situation in mind!

FAILURE TO REACT APPROPRIATELY TO WARNING SIGNS

Both fixation and confirmation bias incline people to dismiss warning signs as aberrations or being irrelevant. Blood pressure monitors sometimes under-read, but equally they can be ignored because of fixation, or dismissed because of confirmation bias.

FAILURE TO COMMUNICATE EFFECTIVELY

Typical signs of overload or confusion are silence, not speaking clearly, asking leading questions, leaving sentences unfinished or questions hanging, asking for a "whatsit", or rambling off the point.

WHEN TAKING OVER

A change of command or shift involves briefing from outgoing to incoming staff. This is a potential source of SA failure for two reasons: first, outgoing staff may have faulty SA; second, the briefing communication process is prone to errors and omissions. In the scenario depicted in the Silva advertisement (see www.safercare.eu/human/), the captain of the *USS Montana* missed this trigger.

THE VAGUE FEELING OF UNEASE

So far we have described things that have been observed from an external viewpoint in team members before incidents occurred, involving the loss of SA. The next point is something that is familiar to us all, but cannot be directly observed, namely the vague feeling of unease. Unconscious cognitive processing occurs in all of us and is rational. Unconscious recognition of patterns containing conflict or threat leads to vague conscious feelings of unease. If someone feels uneasy about a situation, it is likely to be a rational reaction to something being wrong.

Examples of SA checks

The exact mental process of an SA check is hard to explain in words, but it can be shown through the examples in the vignettes in this module.

THE SILVA ADVERTISEMENT (available on the e-learning package at www.safercare.eu/human/)

In this scenario, about the fictional *USS Montana*, Captain Hancock missed the "taking command" SA check. The SA check should have been: *Where are we? Where is he? Are the voice and radar dot coming from the same place?*

THE LOST CAR (Vignette 3.1)

Searching did not have the expected result of finding the car. The SA check could have been: *Is this the right car park? Am I looking for the right car?*

CROHN'S OR APPENDICITIS (Vignette 3.2)

The first time failure of treatment was discussed, an SA check should have been triggered. It would have been an action that did not have the expected result. The SA check should have been: *Is the treatment correct? Is the diagnosis correct?*

WRONG-SIDE EYE SURGERY (Vignette 3.3)

A timely SA check was triggered by a checklist.

Team SA

Among the best known models of SA is that of Endsley, which involves noticing elements of the current situation, understanding the current situation and anticipating future changes.

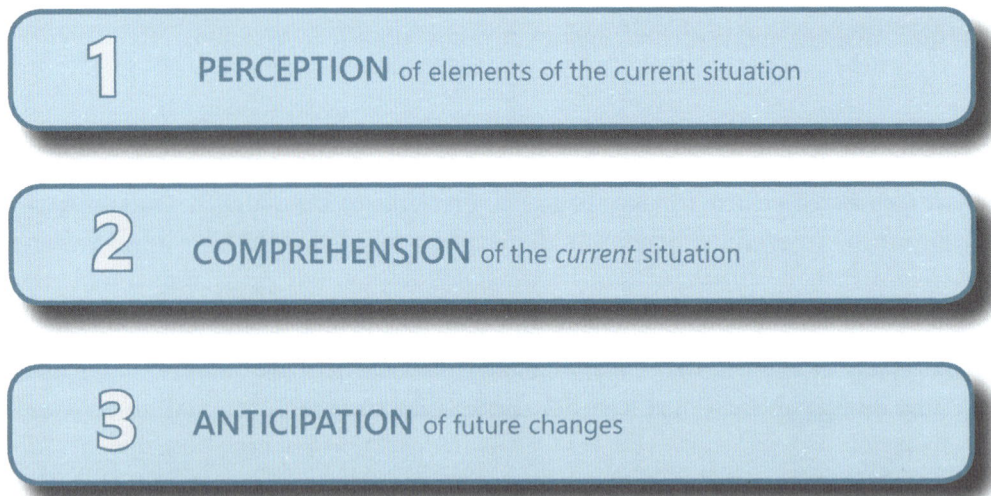

Figure 3.2 *The three levels of situation awareness (SA).*

With experience, we more readily notice things of relevance to our speciality. This is why an experienced coastguard will notice the faintest flare on the horizon, and the mother of a large family looking after any group of children will notice when one disappears. The same applies to understanding and anticipation.

When SA-related mishaps are analysed, the following is observed:

- The majority of mishaps (78% in one aviation study) are caused by failure to notice clues.
- Fewer mishaps (only 17% in the same study) are caused by failure to understand.
- The least mishaps (5%) are caused by failure to anticipate.

Endsley's model implies non-specific appeals to notice more and understand or anticipate better, so it is not much help with our personal SA but it can be applied to other people's.

Everyone's ability to perceive, understand and anticipate will be reduced by lack of knowledge, stress, fixation, distraction and preoccupation. Team members who are preoccupied, for example, underperform at all three steps. If we need to alert them to a situation change it is not good enough to point out the clues. We need to ensure they have understood them and what they mean for the future.

Modes of Team SA failure

Occasionally all team members can lose their SA together. More commonly individual members do, but they can still lead whole teams to fail, even though other members maintain accurate SA. It happens when SA is lost by a senior member or leader. Other members who maintain their SA may remain passive because of their reluctance to challenge authority and because of insecurity in their own judgement.

- **Stage 1**—The first and lowest level is a request for information or clarification.
- **Stage 2**—If this does not resolve the issue, specific conflicting information is pointed out at the second level (remember INCH, as in I Need Clarity Here).

Note that issues rarely go beyond this level, but further levels must be considered because on those rare occasions when they are needed, they are really needed to avoid disaster.

- **Stage 3**—The third level, therefore, is a direct challenge to authority – irrespective of the authority gradient.
- **Stage 4**—The fourth and final level is taking *emergency* action to prevent disaster.

These four steps are encapsulated in the acronym **PACE**.

P robe
A lert
C hallenge
E mergency

Vignette 4.9 Lignocaine and adrenaline?

You are watching a procedure to suture a finger laceration. Local anaesthetic is used. This is done with plane lignocaine – never with lignocaine and adrenaline because adrenaline causes spasm of arteries that can lead to loss of the finger.

Nurses draw up the local anaesthetic from a vial, then put the empty vial in the sharps bin. You think you see red writing on the vial as it goes in the bin, but do not see what it says. Red on a local anaesthetic vial means adrenaline.

What do you do?

PROBE—Maybe take a discrete look into the sharps bin to see if the vial contained adrenalin. Then ask the floor nurse what was in the vial. Does this resolve the problem? If adrenalin is confirmed, or you still do not know, then go to *Alert*.

ALERT—Say to the floor and scrub nurse: "*I thought I saw red on that vial? We do not use that for fingers*". If there is no response, go on to *Challenge*.

CHALLENGE—Say to the surgeon: "*I think that is lignocaine with adrenaline*". If there is still no response (!), proceed to *Emergency*.

EMERGENCY—Have you got time to scrub? Probably not. Pick up that syringe!

Conclusions

At the end of this teaching session, the things to emphasise are not the theoretical models but the lessons that can be realistically applied in the workplace. These are what situation awareness is, how to do an SA check, when to do it, and how to enhance SA in a team with up-gradient and down-gradient communication.

Personality Type

4

Key points for reflection

❶ We each differ in our thoughts, awareness and motivation, and we each have strong and weak areas of observation and understanding.

❷ We tend to judge others according to how they compare to us in our strong areas, and not to realise how they may perform better than us in our weak areas.

❸ If we better understand our personality characteristics, this will give us insights into how we may behave under stress.

❹ There are characteristic errors made by those with differing personality types.

A more detailed understanding of people's strengths, weaknesses, likes and dislikes enables us more effectively to allocate tasks in a way that optimises their efficient completion, as well as the engagement and satisfaction of team members.

Personality typing was an aspect of the ancient theory that the human body was composed of four basic substances, called humours. These four types were associated with the dichotomies of hot/cold and wet/dry, with blood (hot and wet), yellow bile (hot and dry), phlegm (cold and wet) and black bile (cold and dry). In healthy people these four aspects were in balance, and in disease they were out of balance. Fever and sweating were evidence of an excess of blood, which led to the medical profession's past obsession with blood-letting. Hippocrates (460-370 BC) and later Galen (AD 131-200) developed this concept into a theory of four basic temperament traits, each governed by one of the humours.

- Blood was thought to promote a sanguine temperament – extrovert, friendly, talkative, sociable and passionate, but with a tendency to exaggeration and for unreliable reporting.

- Phlegm promotes a phlegmatic temperament – content, kind, and affectionate, but accepting rather than driven and motivated.

- Yellow bile promotes a choleric temperament – ambitious, motivated and energetic, but quick to anger and irritable.

- Black bile promotes a melancholic temperament – thoughtful, quiet and creative, but given to nervousness, anxiety and depression.

This system (see also **Figure 4.1** overpage) remains influential but is not the only one in use.

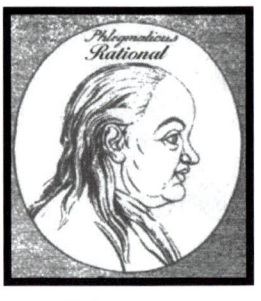 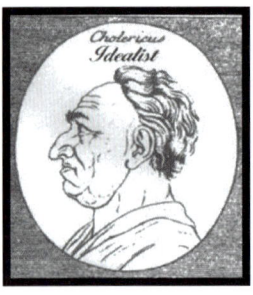 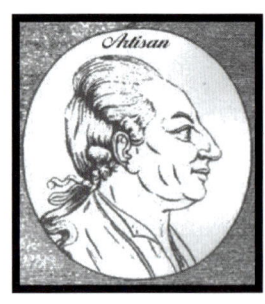 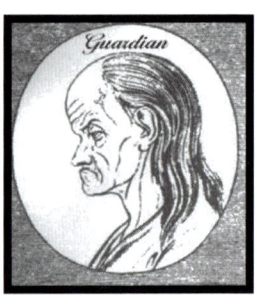

Phlegmaticus
RATIONAL

Cholericus
IDEALIST

Sanguinis
ARTISAN

Melancholius
GUARDIAN

Figure 4.1 *A woodcut depicting the four classical temperaments—phlegmatic, choleric, sanguine and melancholic.*

Type A and type B personalities

These were not devised by psychologists, but by two cardiologists named Friedman and Rosenman who studied the link between people's behaviour and the presence of coronary artery disease. They divided people into Type A and Type B personalities and estimated that Type A personalities had roughly double the risk of developing coronary artery disease than type Bs.

- *Type A* people are aggressive, competitive, ambitious, impatient and highly strung.
- *Type B* people are the opposite – patient, passive and accepting.

The link they proposed to heart disease is controversial.

The Five Factor Model

This is the scientifically rigorous system of personality typing. Data show five groups of characteristics that tend to correlate in any individual. For example, the ease of making friends, the comfort level in a busy social setting and frustration with solitude all tend to occur together in the same person; rarely do we find people who make friends easily but are uncomfortable in a social setting and prefer solitude.

On the other hand laziness occurs together with friendliness no more often than you would expect by chance. The Big Five factors make up the acronym OCEAN.

O penness
C onscientiousness
E xtraversion
A greeableness
N euroticism

Openness to experience

- Inventive and curious versus consistent and cautious.
- Appreciation for *art, emotion, adventure,* unusual ideas, *curiosity* and variety of experience.
- Openness to experience is sometimes labelled *intellect*.

Conscientiousness

- Efficient and organized versus easy-going and careless.
- Tendency to show *self-discipline*, act *dutifully*, and aim for achievement.
- Planned rather than spontaneous behaviour.

Extraversion

- Outgoing and energetic versus solitary and reserved.
- Energy, positive emotions, *surgency*, and the tendency to seek *stimulation* in the company of others.

Agreeableness

- Friendly and compassionate versus cold and unkind.
- Tendency to be *compassionate* and *cooperative* rather than *suspicious* and *antagonistic* towards others.

Neuroticism

- Sensitive and nervous versus secure and confident.
- Tendency to experience unpleasant emotions easily, such as *anger, anxiety, depression* or *vulnerability*.
- Neuroticism is sometimes called *emotional stability*.

Two questionnaires are now widely used to identify the so-called Big Five:

- Neo-Five-Factor Personality Inventory (Neo-PI)
- Hogan Personality Inventory (HPI).

The Neo-PI is used by the National Clinical Assessment service in its psychological assessment of doctors and dentists who get into difficulties.

Jungian models

These originate from C.G. Jung's 1921 book *Psychological Types*. His overall theory was based narrative explanations of thought, and tested using introspection and anecdotal personal observations on other people. Jung was an astute observer whose practice as a psychotherapist gave him access to the intimate details of other people's thoughts.

Jung proposed two attitudes and four functions (two *Perceiving* and two *Judging*):

- **Attitudes (2)**
  Extroversion (E)
  Introversion (I)

- **Functions (4)**
  Perceiving—Sensation (S) and iNtuition (N)
  Judging—Thinking (T) and Feeling (F)

These are shown in his model of personality (**Figure 4.2**).

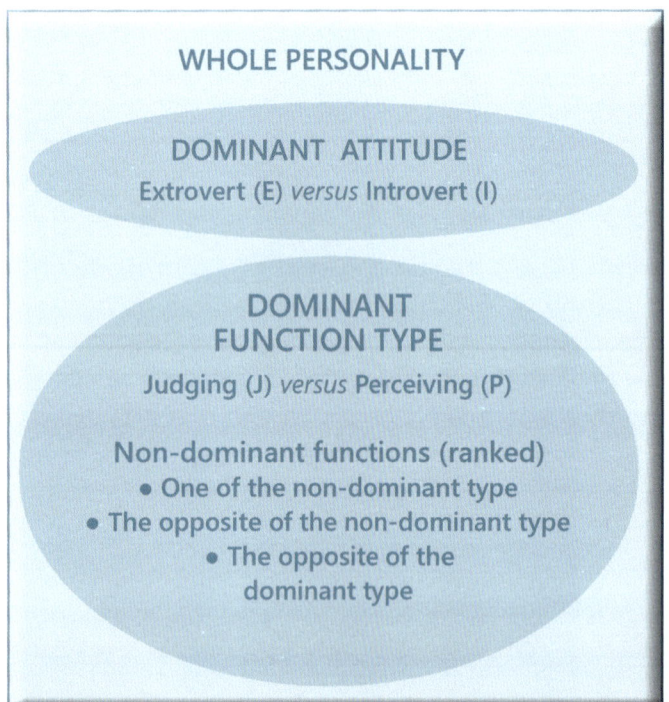
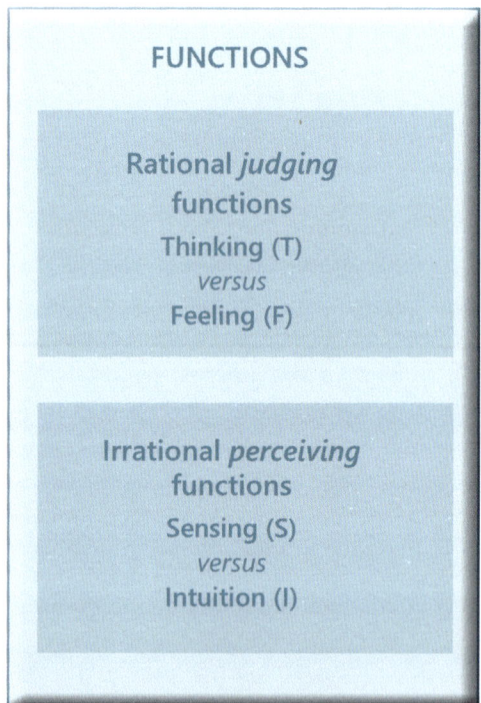

Figure 4.2 *Carl Jung's model of personality.*

Jung believed that personality type is fixed from early childhood throughout life. Different personality types have good and bad features. In everyday life we present an *affected persona* that attempts to conceal the shortcomings of our personality, while showing the strengths. However, maintaining a different persona from our personality requires effort. Our mental capacity is limited and when we are under stress our behaviour will revert to that native of our personality. This is known as *reversion to type*.

We discuss two Jungian systems below. They are both part of commercial and popular psychology but they have little weight in academic psychology.

Myers–Briggs Type Indicator (MBTI)

This is an adaptation of Jung's system and it is the market leader in the commercial exploitation of personality typing, where its use and much of the information about it are controlled by the company.

The MTBI uses these terms for Jung's four dichotomies:

E = Extrovert	vs	I = Introvert
S = Sensing	vs	N = iNtuitive
T = Thinking	vs	F = Feeling
J = Judging	vs	P = Perceiving

Formal use involves answering a series of forced questions (i.e you are asked not to leave any answers blank) in a session with an approved trainer. Informal use involves describing what is meant by the four dichotomies and then asking respondents to classify themselves. The result is one of 16 combinations of letters (e.g. INTP).

Keirsey Temperament Sorter (KTS)

The American psychologist, Keirsey, uses Jung's dichotomies in a hierarchical system comprising four main temperaments, eight roles and sixteen role variants. We have chosen his model, the Keirsey Temperament Sorter or KTS, as the basis of this module and thus will describe it in some detail.

Table 4.1 *The KTS personality classification system*

	Temperament	Role	Role variant
SENSING	Guardian (SJ)	Administrator (STJ)	Supervisor (ESTJ)
			Inspector (ISTJ)
		Conservator (SFJ)	Provider (ESFJ)
			Protector (ISFJ)
	Artisan (SP)	Operator (STP)	Promotor (ESTP)
			Crafter (ISTP)
		Entertainer (SFP)	Performer (ESFP)
			Composer (ISFP)
INTUITIVE	Idealist (NF)	Mentor (NFJ)	Teacher (ENFJ)
			Counsellor (INFJ)
		Advocate (NFP)	Champion ENFP)
			Healer (INFP)
	Rational (NT)	Coordinator (NTJ)	Field-marshall (ENTJ)
			Mastermind (INTJ)
		Engineer (NTP)	Inventor (ENTP)
			Architect (INTP)

Keirsey's interpretation of the dichotomies

DICHOTOMY 1—THOUGHT
Sensing vs iNtuitive (S–N)

The top dichotomy in the hierarchy is better described as *observing detail* versus *deriving general principles*. We have a mental model of ourselves and our environment. Building this model involves two things, sensing our environment and deriving general principles from the sensed information to allow us to determine things we cannot sense, such as what we cannot see or what will happen in the future. We do both, but not equally.

- **Sensing**—Around 75% of people are Sensing. Their mental model is primarily built on experiences, including sights, taste and sounds, and they notice these easily and without effort. They do as much general principle derivation as they need to, but no more, because it does not come easily to them. Under pressure they tend to prioritise gathering and assessing this data over the general task in hand. They can fail to see the wood for the trees.

- **Intuitive**—A minority of people are Intuitive. For them, deriving general principles comes easily and without effort, but sensing does not. They sense only what they need to inform the development of the general principles that occupy most of their thought. They conceptualise issues and problems through general principles, rather than building up a picture from observation of data and detail. They are specifically observant of things that allow them to discriminate between different possible theories or scenarios. They appreciate systems, elegant logical arguments and debates between possible explanations of what is observed. They can jump to conclusions.

DICHOTOMY 2—ORDER
Judging vs Perceiving (J–P)

This dichotomy relates to how we deal with information and observations. For those with a preference for data and detail (sensors), this is the next most important dichotomy. It refers to a need for order.

- **Judging**—Judging people seek order in what they do. They are schedulers who prefer organised lives with tasks completed one by one. They resist changes they see as unnecessary. They can appear as rigid and inflexible.

- **Perceiving**—Perceiving people do not need order and they resist it when externally imposed. They keep several tasks going at once, flitting from one to another as the need arises – the need often being a looming deadline! They like to leave options open in case things change. They become bored with routine and seek novelty out of curiosity. They are seen by judging people as chaotic and disorganised, but cope well with change and are flexible and adaptable. They can appear to be indecisive.

This dichotomy can lead to conflict between people of opposite types. Perceivers readily resent judging colleagues or bosses because they view them as rigid, inflexible and controlling; Judgers view perceivers as disorganised and chaotic.

DICHOTOMY 3—FEELINGS
Thinking vs Feeling (T–F)

This refers to introspection, and is the second dichotomy to apply when classifying intuitives.

- **Thinkers**—Thinkers favour thought in logic, geometric space and time, that is expressible in language, over feelings. They do not trust their feelings and particularly dislike feelings that conflict with reason. Thinkers do not like to show emotion and are inclined to embarrassment by displays of feeling in others. They make logical, analytical decisions. They may then give some thought to the likely effect of their decision on others, or may not particularly if they are under stress. If they do express feelings under stress, they may do this in a less skilled and unrestrained manner.

- **Feelers**—Feelers are the opposite. They think in terms of core values, morality and meaning. They trust their feelings and attend to them. They do not have the thinkers' inhibitions about showing emotions or allowing them to influence what they say and do. They make decisions based on their effect on themselves and others and may then give some thought to whether the decision makes any sense, or may not particularly if under stress.

Like Judging versus Perceiving, this dichotomy can lead to conflict between people of opposite types. Thinkers view feelers as illogical and inconsistent; Feelers view thinkers as insensitive and cold – even cruel.

DICHOTOMY 4—OTHER PEOPLE
Extroversion vs Introversion (E–I)

This refers to dealing with other people, and how sociable someone is.

- **Extroverts**—Extroverts prefer to relax with others and to interact with others. They are refreshed by social interaction. Under pressure or stress they tend to become talkative. They rapidly become frustrated and lonely with solitude.

- **Introverts**—Introverts prefer to keep their thoughts and feelings private. They need to spend time alone or with just a few close associates, to re-energise, relax, and organise their thoughts. They are fatigued by social interaction. Under pressure or stress they tend to become silent.

Jung and the MBTI both discuss this dichotomy first, but Keirsey leaves it to last because he considers it to be the least important one. This is because, unlike the others, its value in predicting how people behave goes no further than the dichotomy itself. Thus, being an extrovert says nothing more about someone than when they are in contact with other people they are extroverted.

Structure of the KTS

The structure of the KTS is shown in **Table 4.1**. The central idea is that of four temperaments, which are analogous to Galen's four-way classification system. People of different temperaments are quite different from each other, whereas different roles and role variants within the same temperament are quite similar. **Table 4.2** shows some of the different traits of the four temperaments.

Table 4.2 *The KTS temperament types*

Personality trait	SENSOR TEMPERAMENT		INTUITIVE TEMPERAMENT	
	Guardian (SJ)	Artisan (SP)	Idealist (NF)	Rational (NT)
Education	Commerce	Artefacts	Humanities	Science
Aptitude	Logistics	Tactics	Diplomacy	Strategy
Attitude	Stoical	Hedonistic	Altruistic	Pragmatic
Future Views	Pessimistic	Optimistic	Credulous	Sceptical
Looks For ...	Security	Stimulation	Identity	Knowledge
Most Values ...	Gratitude	Generosity	Recognition	Deference
Preoccupied With ...	Morality	Techniques	Morale	Technology
Vocation	Material	Equipment	Personnel	Systems
Vices	Controlling	Feckless	Gullible	Cruel
Virtues	Respectable	Resolute	Authentic	Adaptable
Wants To Be ...	Dependable	Artistic	Empathic	Ingenious
Tends To Be ...	Concerned	Excited	Enthusiastic	Calm
Trusts	Authority	Impulse	Intuition	Reason
Longs For ...	Belonging	Impact	Romance	Achievement

Guardian temperaments (SJ)

Guardians favour observation over introspection and order over novelty. Jung and the MBTI classify them as SJ and Galen as melancholic, being solemn and prepared for the worst.

Their strength is in responsibility. They are the pillars of society, ensuring things run smoothly, supplies are available, everyone's needs are met, transport runs on time, shops remain supplied, staff turn up to work and do what they should. They are diligent and reliable. They are often asked to help out and their sense of responsibility makes it difficult for them to decline a request. Consequently they tend to end up over-worked and over-committed socially, working long hours for their employers and helping out with school functions, charitable events, and voluntary work in their spare time. Logistics is the skill they have the greatest aptitude for (compared to tactics for the Artisans, strategy for the Rationals and diplomacy for the Idealists). Logistics is about making material goods and services available where and when they are needed. Their weakness is strategy with tactics and diplomacy in between.

They respect authority, believe in hierarchical structures of authority and trust people in authority or recognised experts. They see rules as being there for a purpose; even if they do not fully understand what that purpose is (they assume someone else does and is prepared to trust them). Guardians expend their own time and effort to create and enforce the rules that ensure societies and organisations run smoothly. They are good at making wise and effective rules that benefit everyone. They have a strong moral sense of right and wrong and of personal duty to those around them. They are concerned about numerous social, professional, family or environmental issues and take a stoical outlook, particularly in areas such as hard work and saving. They feel a duty of service – not so much for joy as for obligation. They need to feel respectable.

Self-confidence can be a problem for Guardians who are averse to showing off. They are proud of, and collect, awards and qualifications in the pursuit of respectability. They tend to be pessimistic about the future, and believe in "Murphy's Law" – that is, whatever can go wrong will (and adding "It will be my fault if I let it"). Their speech is of concrete things like jobs, housing, credit, debt and prices rather than abstractions and generalisations. In conversation they change topic easily by association, so the price of petrol may prompt a change to types of car (whereas for other temperament types it would more likely prompt discussion of the factors influencing price). This ability to cover wide ranges of subjects makes Guardians good at holding everyone's interest. They also have impressive memory for socially important facts. They easily remember names, faces, family ties, whose children are doing what, and so on, giving them the best social skills of all the temperaments. They are cooperative for common goals which makes them natural team players.

Guardians like routine and resist change for its own sake. They trust tradition and tend to think things are not as good as they used to be. They are people of regular habits, who follow the same routines each day. They value durable items like heirlooms, collections and family photographs. They do not like to see old building demolished or old trees cut down. They like to see themselves as beneficent to others, particularly when it comes to food, clothing, shelter and transport. They are good hosts but get upset if they are not appreciated and they like to receive offers of help even though they are reluctant to accept them. They prize gratitude and find it galling when others exploit them without giving any (but of all temperaments, they are the least able to ask for it).

Furthermore, the tasks they take on tend to be thankless. If a Guardian is hosting dinner party, they will ensure the supplies are available, will set the table and wash up (often helped by Guardian guests), and attend to the guests, to make sure they are all are provided for and that no-one is left out (they will be quick to notice if anyone is feeling left out and take corrective action). These efforts are essential for a successful evening but only attract attention when they are not done, rather than when they are.

Artisan temperaments (SP)

Artisans are sensing and perceiving and are Galen's sanguine temperament. They think and communicate in vivid and closely observed detail, focusing on the here and now and their immediate environment rather than on generalisations or principles.

They are interested in experiencing things, particularly if they are novel or different. When considering a fine car they are interested in its shape and colour, its smell, acceleration and handling. Other temperaments are more interested in its inner workings. Artisans get bored with routine tasks and seek change out of curiosity. They excel in short-term reactive situations such as entertainment, emergency responses and team tactics. Of the four types they have the best ability to sense and exploit their immediate environment – this is called tactical intelligence. They are not so good at long-term strategic planning and having sensitivity to other people's feelings, and have little interest in morality or morale.

Their educational interests are in creative arts and crafts. These are not high educational priorities in the western world and Artisans are often frustrated and distracted and tend to under-achieve at school. Their learning interest is in perfecting skills, be they musical, artistic, technical or dramatic. They are attracted to instruments and machines, not because of their workings but because of what they do to their environment and the Artisan's desire to experience and master them. They want to drive the motorcycle, fly the plane, shoot the arrow, and wield the mallet and chisel. These properties combine to make them the greatest of athletes, artists, sculptors and cooks.

The Artisan's attitude to the present is hedonistic; they do things "for the fun of it" and see no point in doing something they do not have to do if there is no enjoyment in it. They are optimistic about the short-term future and do not worry about the long-term. Compared to other temperaments, they have a casual, happy-go-lucky attitude to life that can lead them into trouble and tends towards boom and bust rather than stability. They may be cynical and distrustful about the motives of other people. They want to see themselves as creative, accomplished and graceful in action. Their keenest embarrassment is in being dull, unskilled or clumsy. They want to be bold and adventurous, and feel guilty about cowardice or demurring adventure. They are the great risk-takers. They also see themselves as being adaptable to changing circumstances and good in a crisis. They frequently act on impulse (including being impulsively generous). Their longing is to create a social or cultural impact, to be noticed and to attract wide attention.

Intuitive temperaments

Three of the dichotomies in the KTS divide the population into roughly equal groups. The exception is Sensing versus Intuitive. Sensors outnumber Intuitives, who make up 15–25% of the population, and this has a bearing on how they develop. The thought processes of Sensors and Intuitives can be inaccessible to each other. Sensors find themselves surrounded by other Sensors, with the occasional misfit they do not understand. Intuitives find themselves surrounded by Sensors who they do not understand, with the occasional soul-mate. These develop into life-long feelings of inclusion for the Sensors, Artisans and Guardians, but detachment for the Intuitives, Idealists and Rationals.

IDEALISTS (NF)

The Intuitive Feelers are Galen's cholerics. Idealists talk not of what they observe, but of what is in their minds. They talk of strong feelings, love, hate, empathy and passion, symbols, fantasies and meanings. They are highly imaginative and move rapidly from the particular to the general, the general being abstract moralities and feelings. They are sensitive to nuance and meaning, making them the best at mind-reading and reading between the lines. They have a desire to connect disparate ideas and concepts into a coherent whole. They are given to exaggeration and hyperbole. The meal that the Rational finds adequate, the Idealist finds exquisite. They dream of perfect interpersonal relationships and their first instinct is to promote those things ahead of achieving material goals. They particularly dislike fighting in any form and can be deeply hurt by callous criticism. Their sensitivity to others, reluctance to upset, avoidance of conflict and keenness to please makes diplomacy their strong suit. They are altruistic, believing self-service is bad and service to others is good. They believe there is good in everyone and feel driven to find it. Idealists are typically drawn to humanities and social sciences rather than hard sciences or commerce, and they are not great with technology. They prefer working with words and people to tools and things. They are pre-occupied with the morale of those around them, unlike the guardians who are preoccupied with the comfort and physical needs of those around them. They choose careers that involve teaching, caring, and guiding people. Idealists want to be benevolent towards people, things and the earth. They suppress feelings of malice, revenge, hatred or cruelty. They want to be genuine and authentic, with no false façade. More than other temperaments, idealists are self-conscious, and feel the eyes of others on them. They are highly sensitive to the way they are judged by others. They feel inadequate and lose self-confidence if they give a false impression of themselves and fear others are able to look straight through their contrived façade.

Idealists are credulous and given to metaphysical and religious beliefs. They easily believe in things and causes, especially if they have faith in leading figures, and they can develop fixed ideas from which logical reasoning will not shake them. Idealists are emotional and usually positive so they like enthusiasm, but when they are frustrated or treated harshly they show Galen's choleric properties of quickness to anger.

Idealists seek inner meaning and a sense of personal identity, or finding themselves, so much so that they have been called the identity seeking personality (note seeking, not finding!). They can be incurable romantics and appreciate recognition for who they are rather than the roles they must play in society. They can go through life feeling misunderstood.

RATIONALS (NT)

Introspective Thinkers are Galen's phlegmatics, whom he described as not being easily excited to emotion or action, calm, apathetic, composed, distant and detached. Keirsey's corresponding temperament is the Rational. Rationals spend much of their lives in abstract thought, thinking in three-dimensional space, time, logical relationships, causes and effects. They think more prominently in language and less in feelings, desires and impressions than other temperaments. They become highly practised at this and have the best ability of all types to comprehend the workings of the physical world and to predict the results of actions. They prefer to think rather than act, and when addressing a task they will give thought to how the task can be done to achieve maximum effect for minimum effort. This makes them the most efficient temperament in use of time and resources. They like being asked to devise, implement or explain complex systems; preferably all three together. They are adaptable and tolerant, judging ideas and people on their merits alone.

They talk of what is imagined, not of what is seen, and their use of language is precise. They do not exaggerate and they speak in terms of possible, probable, consistent with – rarely in terms of facts or proof. They are economical with words and tend not to elaborate, assuming others will understand as they do. Others may not follow them, however, and Rationals are prone to losing their audience and becoming impatient with other people's "stupidity". They are highly curious and seek knowledge for its own sake. They are sceptical about the ideas and claims of others.

A particular aspect of their temperament is their yearning for achievement, unlike the "drivers" of the other temperaments (belonging for Guardians; making an impact for Artisans; romance for Idealists). They are drawn to the study of systems in science and mathematics. Today's largely clerical primary-school curriculum bores them and they tend to under-perform at basic literacy, gaining success in secondary school and further education where their favoured subjects are available to study. They trust reason fully, intuition rarely, impulse rarely, and external authority never. Rules and morals are of secondary importance if they cannot be used to get results.

Rationals are not socially or politically correct, but neither are they given to snobbishness or prejudice and they do not care for status, position, qualifications, reputation, authority, prestige or other badges of social acceptability. They are autonomous and ignore any law or instruction that does not make sense to them. Ideas must stand on their own merit; authority, title or reputation count for little. This lack of respect for authority can lead to conflict. Rationals are risk-takers, but for different reasons than Artisans.

Most people's view of the risk of something bad happening is based on how bad it would be if it happened – and only secondarily on how likely it is to happen. The Rational's view is based in equal measure on the severity of the risk and the statistical probability of it happening. This makes them inclined to ignore the risk of disaster if they see it as being highly improbable, and their ability accurately to judge such probabilities is greater than that of other types. They like to remain calm, particularly under stress and if they cannot keep calm they will try not to let it show. Of all the temperaments they are the most critical of their own abilities, but they allow no external criticism that is not carefully measured and warranted. Criticism that they see as unjust or inaccurate can turn them into dangerous enemies, harbouring secret resentments for years and plotting efficient, vindictive revenge.

Problems with Jungian classification systems

Several criticisms are applied to the Jungian systems covered here, namely the MBTI and KTS.

Test–retest reliability

This refers to how well two tests done on the same person agree with one another. For the MBTI, agreement varies from just over 80% to under 40%, and this agreement declines when there is a greater time interval between the two tests. Contrary to Jung's beliefs, this finding suggests that such tests are not measuring unchanging life-long characteristics.

Dichotomy

A characteristic like extroversion is not an all-or-none phenomenon; rather it forms a continuous spectrum from extreme extroversion at one end to extreme introversion at the other. Modelling this as a *dichotomy* is not entirely satisfactory because it fails to distinguish between the extreme case whose personality is dominated by that one trait alone, and the more typical, intermediate case.

Evidence base

There are three ways to generate evidence in personality studies:

    (i) one-to-one case studies,
    (ii) questionnaires from large numbers of respondents, and
    (iii) laboratory experiments.

All have their strengths and weaknesses. However, Jungian systems are based on only one of these, that is one-to-one case studies. This method has the advantage of providing indepth detailed analysis, but the disadvantages of subjectivity, interobserver variation and thus limited repeatability.

Mainstream psychology favours systems that are informed by repeatable lines if evidence, such as the Five Factor model and neo-PI. The problem of these is that they do not use one-to-one evidence at all, so they lack the indepth narrative obtained through Jungian systems.

Horoscope effect

Jungian classification systems are likened to fortune-telling – and for good reason. Both the MTBI and the KTS start by asking questions and then use a combination of tautology with the answers to those questions, non-specific extrapolation, and subtle flattery (particularly the MBTI) in order to make their predictions sound credible. A critical point is about tautological versus non-tautological prediction. The main feature of people's personalities is their consistency over time; this means that tautological prediction is generally pretty accurate. If somebody reports being tidy, they are likely to have a tidy desk and a tidy bedroom for many years in the future. This is a tautological prediction because it predicts behaviour that is the same as the behaviour that has been reported. Non-tautological predictions are those such as Sensing Judgers respect authority, or Intuitive Thinkers do not respect authority. Non-tautological predictions are less accurate than tautological ones. The wider the gap between what has been reported and what is being claimed, the less reliable the predictions are.

Conclusions

People's personality types differ more than we expect from cursory observations. Understanding these differences helps us work with people more efficiently, distributing tasks and roles to those who are best at them. This allows tasks to be completed to a higher standard and individual's to work with less stress and greater satisfaction.

Team Working

Key points for reflection

❶ Groups are just collections of individual people, whereas teams optimise their members' deployment to make the whole better than the sum of the individuals.

❷ For teams to be optimal, communication, team-member development and member deployment need to be undertaken effectively.

Team-working refers to the difference between the overall effectiveness of a team and the sum of the effectiveness of its individual members:

- Group-working involves individuals coming together to perform a task or achieve a target. This group is only as effective as the sum of its members.
- Team-working involves motivating and coordinating each member's strengths and weaknesses to maximise the team's effectiveness as a whole. The team is more effective than the sum of its members.

Workplaces default to group-working. To achieve team-working requires a vision, with a leader who is able to develop that vision within the team as well as the ability of all the team-members to align their personal objectives with those of the team as a whole. Conflicting opinions are to be expected, and resolution, if handled skilfully, will enhance the strength of the team.

Table 5.1 *Teams versus groups*

Teams	Groups
■ Decision by consensus	■ Decisions often not made
■ Disagreements discussed and resolved	■ Unresolved disagreements
■ Objectives well understood and agreed by members	■ Objectives often not agreed
■ All members contribute ideas	■ Personal feelings often hidden
■ Frequent team self examination	■ Discussions avoided regarding group functioning
■ Members understand their roles	■ Individuals protect their roles
■ Share leadership on as-needed basis	■ Leadership appointed

Healthcare perspective

The UK's National Health Service is the world's seventh largest employer with 1.4 million workers. Its size and multiple hierarchies mean that NHS teams are often indistinct and constantly changing.

Analysis by team inventory shows that most of the time NHS staff work as groups rather than teams, an observation that will surprise few people; poor team-working is a ubiquitous conclusion of investigations into adverse events.

Healthcare is behind other industries with respect to deploying team-work training and it is still reliant on imported methods from fields such as aviation in which training is widely implemented but little robust evidence of its benefit has been produced.

Some evidence has been gathered within the strongly evidence-based culture of healthcare (summarised below) but lack of evidence of any benefit remains a limitation.

Possible benefits of effective team-work suggested by the evidence

Benefits for patients

- Reduction in mortality (by 5%)
- Reduction in errors by positive contribution to performance
- Reduction in patient time in hospital (shown to save more money than the cost of running the teams)
- Improvement in service provision by streamlining services
- Enhancement in patient satisfaction
- Improved decision-making

Benefits for staff

- Decrease in sickness rates within the team (doctors in poor teams have an almost two-fold increase in sickness rates)
- Better decision-making
- Increased motivation
- Increased well-being (21% of staff in real teams report above-threshold stress levels compared to 30% of staff in loose teams or groups and 35% of staff in no teams)

In summary

Although it is not easy to prove, it is widely believed that effective teams result in:

- Improved patient outcomes
- Reduced hospital stays and costs
- Improved working lives of staff.

Whatever the science involved, there is no doubt about the politics of team-working. The report from the Bristol paediatric heart surgery inquiry (the Kennedy report) made numerous references to the dangers of ineffective team-working, including this quote:

> " ... it should be the norm for surgical teams (the surgeon, anaesthetist, theatre nurses, operating department assistants) to have time together and with other teams, such as those in the ITU, to review and develop their performance as a team."

Unlike other scandals and disasters, there was no single event or individual behind the failings of the Bristol hospital and the reasons it came to public consciousness did not relate to how uniquely bad the situation was, but to a coincidence of other circumstances.

1. A powerful outcome measure

Paediatric heart surgery was the speciality involved and even in the best of hands this specialty has a substantial mortality. This has two consequences: first, paediatric deaths are highly emotive and attract more public interest than the equivalent numbers of adult deaths; second, performance can be easily and objectively measured.

2. The presence of a whistle-blower

Dr Stephen Bolsin was appointed as a consultant anaesthetist at the hospital in 1989. He noted the high mortality, but unlike other people was prepared to knowingly sacrifice his professional popularity (and his job) in order to correct the situation.

Without these two factors, it is probable that this situation would have gone on unchallenged. The relevance of this is that the failings of the hospital were – and are -- not restricted to that unit at that time! They are equally applicable to numerous other units in other specialties that have avoided the coincidence of a powerful outcome measure and the presence of a whistle-blower. Not surprisingly, the Kennedy report makes eerily familiar reading to other healthcare professionals.

The origin of the team approach

The study of team-working dates from the 1920s and 1930s when there was a fashion in the USA for scientific management, involving time-and-motion experiments in which things like workplace lighting, temperature, piped music, break patterns and pay systems were varied, and their effect on productivity was observed.

The Western Electric Company conducted a study on lighting at their Hawthorne plant and found that the lighting level made no difference to the productivity of their workers, but when the factory was being studied they found that productivity improved. When the study ended, productivity fell back to previous levels.

This effect was studied further in the bank-wiring room which is described overpage.

The bank-wiring room

Bank wiring involved connecting wires to banks of terminals on telephone equipment. For this experiment, a special room was set up for this purpose. There were fourteen workers in the room: nine wirers (to install the wires), three solderers (to solder the connections) and two inspectors. An observer was also in the room. Initially the workers would not talk freely when the observer was within earshot, but after three weeks their normal behaviours resumed. Analysis showed that the most significant factor in the effectiveness of the bank-wiring room was the building of a sense of group identity, and a feeling of social support and cohesion that came with increased interaction between the workers. This was promoted by a number of factors. These are:

WHEN THE MANAGER—
- had a personal interest in each person's achievements
- took pride in the record of the group
- helped the group set its own conditions of work
- faithfully posted feedback on members performance.

WHEN THE GROUP—
- took pride in its own achievements and had the satisfaction of outsiders showing interest in what they did
- did not feel they were being pressured to change
- was consulted before changes were made
- developed a sense of confidence and candour.

These conditions can still be used to judge the effectiveness of any team in the twenty-first century.

Team motivation

Without productive motivation we default to other motives like fear, greed, sloth, wrath, envy and pride. Achieving constructive motivation is a central part of team-working. Various methods can help achieve it as described below in turn.

Buy-in

Team members are motivated if they agree that the team's goals are worthwhile, so the team members must know what they are and why they matter, with clear explanations of where their own task fits in and why their own role is important.

The UK NHS is particularly prone to one issue that affects "buy in", that is the conflict between political and technical motivation.

- *Political motivation* leads personnel to do things that improve the impression of the NHS's performance to the wider electorate.

- *Technical motivation* leads personnel to reduce the impact of disease on individual patients, as far as possible.

These motivations often come into conflict. Front-line staff tend to be technically motivated, while administrators and managers tend to be politically motivated. Politically motivated people can see technically motivated people as narrow and naive, while technically motivated people can see politically motivated people as expedient and self-serving. Neither group is wholly right or wholly wrong.

The way to address the problem is for both sides to understand the other's position. If you are on one side of such a conflict, make a conscious effort to understand the other side's point of view before explaining your own – rather than the other way round.

Appreciation

Team members will be better motivated if their efforts are appreciated. People feel appreciated when they are involved in tasks and decisions that are appropriate to their experience and skills.

Skill deployment

There is a close relationship between what we are good at and what we like doing. Optimal team-working involves distributing tasks in a team so that each member is given the tasks that best match their skills. This has the obvious advantage that tasks given to people who are good at them will be done well, but also it benefits the morale of the whole team. People are better motivated when they are doing something they are good at and enjoy, and they are more likely to be appreciated and easier to "buy in". It takes time for team members to get to know what each another is good at, but the process can be speeded up by encouraging discussion about what tasks need to be done and who would like to do them. There are, of course, always routine, repetitive or tedious tasks that are not popular with anyone. Boredom and consequent demotivation can be mitigated by variation, so that individual team members do not always end up doing the same thing, but instead change roles within their capabilities. Several attempts have been made to classify the roles people take in teams. The *Belbin Team Inventory* is one of the better known ones and is summarised below.

Role in team	Description of role
Plant	A creative generator of ideas
Resource investigator	Gets the necessary resources from outside the team
Coordinator	Overall coordinator or tasks
Shaper	Committed to achieving the team's goal and motivates others to do so
Monitor–evaluator	Detached and unbiased logical observer and judge of what is going on in the team
Team-worker	Diplomat who aids understanding, defuses aggression and resolves conflict
Implementer	Takes the suggestions of others and acts on them
Completer–finisher	A perfectionist who ensures all is as it should be
Specialist	Brings a details knowledge of the subject at hand, but tends to be disinterested in other things

Skill development

People get familiar with the tasks they do regularly, so deployment affects the skills they develop. One healthcare issue is the continuity of service through changes in team membership. Many departments contain leading specialists and consequently enjoy reputations for excellence. Too often, however, these departmental reputations collapse when key individuals retire or move on.

Another issue concerns the provision of emergency services. This requires twenty-four-hour on-call teams with members working in shifts. A single individual cannot provide such a service alone. These issues require development of team skills, whereby members work together on particularly demanding tasks, partly to make the task easier and safer, but also to share skill development.

Use of time

If tasks were always given to those who are best at them, senior team members would end up busier and more stressed than the junior members. If a junior (or less able) team member is under-occupied, then identifying an area in which to develop his or her skills will improve their engagement with the team.

Optimal deployment of time and skills requires every team member to have a close working knowledge of the other team members. This is best done by the team and the immediate team leader. Unfortunately it is often done by remote managers, so it is rarely achieved in practice.

Briefings

Team briefings occur at an allocated time at the start of the day or shift, enabling the team to meet and prepare themselves. It is more than an exchange of information. It also serves to lower authority or power and distance gradients, and therefore empowers more junior team members to bring up concerns or clarify uncertainties.

Mini-briefs are carried out throughout the day to alert team members to alterations of plans or changes of situations and to help keep common and accurate situation awareness.

Process improvement

Process improvement refers to a team's performance being at least maintained, and ideally improving over time. An important tool in process improvement is feedback whereby team members discuss any problems that have arisen in a situation (and might be avoided in the future) as well as everything that went well (and could be repeated in the future).

Many industries use debriefing, which are formal sessions set aside at the end of tasks or shifts for feedback. In many healthcare settings, such as operating theatres, debriefing meetings are not practicable because the shifts or tasks of individual team members finish at different times and there is no specific time when everyone is available at once.

Teams that use regular feedback outperform teams that do not, and even if debriefing is not practical then feedback should still be elicited and applied. This can be done using "hot debriefs" in which any issue – positive or negative – is discussed at the first available opportunity after it occurs.

In the following vignette, hot debriefing enabled an accurate, blame-free, decisive analysis. It is doubtful that enough detail of the checking process would have been retained had the usual investigative processes been followed, without a hot debriefing.

> **Vignette 5.3   More wrong-side surgery**
>
> A surgery department had an apparently watertight checking system to prevent wrong-side errors. A junior surgeon was operating on a patient. Shortly after the operation had begun – on the wrong side – the senior surgeon came into the theatre and recognised the error. The operation was immediately halted. Members of the team were asked about what happened, with no implications of blame. A number of causative factors emerged, the principal one being that the checks had been followed but the read-back system had used leading questions, including: "This is the right side, isn't it?" rather than "What is the intended side?"

The checking system was changed accordingly. For the patient, the harm was limited to an extra scar, about which they were graciously forgiving!

Team-work training systems

The aviation industry has taken a lead in human factors skills and its current training system is called NOTECHS (Non-Technical Skills). This uses a behavioural marker system to describe human interaction in four categories:

- Two *cognitive* categories: situation awareness and decision making.
- Two *social* categories: leadership and team-working.

The NOTECHS category of team-work is also referred to as communication and cooperation. It is divided into four elements, each of which has observable and teachable behaviours – both positive and negative (see **Table 5.2**).

Table 5.3 The NOTECH category of team-work

Team function	Traits and roles
Team building/maintaining	■ Relaxed ■ Supportive ■ Open ■ Inclusive ■ Polite ■ Friendly ■ Uses humour: ■ Does not compete
Support of others	■ Helps others ■ Offers assistance ■ Gives feedback
Understanding team needs	■ Listens to others ■ Recognizes ability of team ■ Considers condition of others ■ Gives personal feedback
Conflict solving	■ Keeps calm in conflicts ■ Suggests conflict solutions ■ Concentrates on what is right

Safer Care: Human Factors for Healthcare

With this system, an experienced observer can pinpoint which elements of team-work are effective or ineffective. The system has been extrapolated and developed for health care, such as the:

- Non-Technical Skills for Surgeons (NOTTS)
- Anaesthetists' Non-Technical Skills (ANTS)
- Oxford NOTECHS (ON)
- Team Self-Review (TSR)

The generic example of the team-working category of a NOTECH system in **Table 5.3** has been used successfully to train teams in operating theatres. The NOTECH system is a great help in assessing team-work skills, but it is short-term in its scope. **Table 5.3** shows that motivation, skill development, skill deployment, use of time and process improvement are missing, and these omissions reflect the origin of the system that was used by independent observers of flight-deck behaviour among airline crew over periods of a few hours.

> Communication + Cooperation = Teamwork

Error management

This is a key concept in human factors management that has relevance to leadership, system design, stress management and situation awareness – as well as team-working. It is included in this module but could equally have been considered in the context of these other subjects, or on its own. That concept is that human error is unavoidable and must be *managed* as opposed to *prevented*.

Swiss Cheese model

James Reason of Manchester University proposed the Swiss Cheese model, in which an organisation's defence against errors can be modelled as slices of cheese containing randomly placed holes. When the holes in several slices line up, errors can occur (**Figure 5.1**).

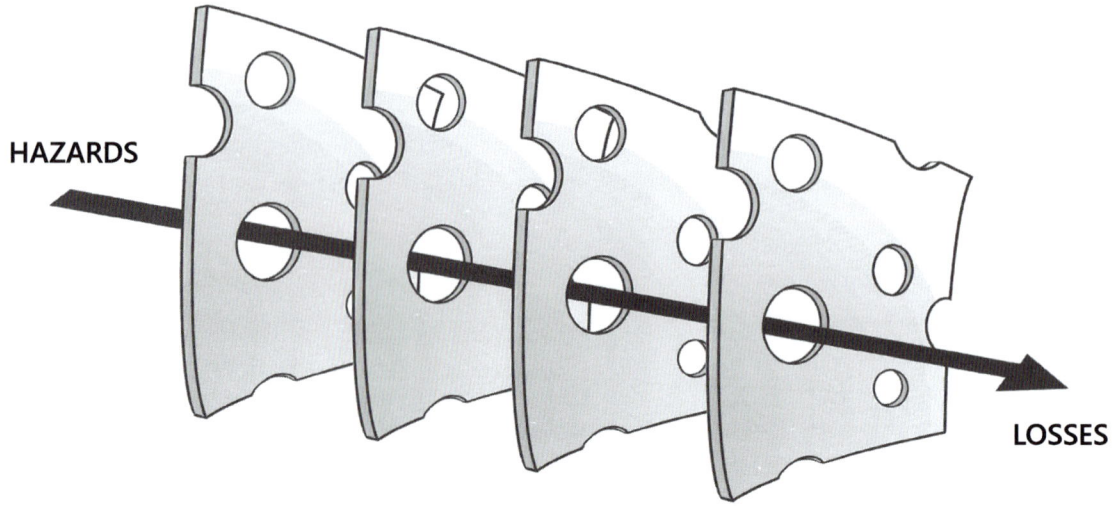

Figure 5.1 *The Swiss cheese model.*

Protection in the Swiss Cheese model is seen as a series of barriers, each with its own weaknesses, which vary in place and size. Some of them are avoidable lapses or errors; some are unavoidable hazards. Failures happen when weaknesses in all the barriers line up and result in a "trajectory of accident opportunity". This fits well with experience, where a series of errors are generally involved in any accident and most potential accidents are caught in the earlier stages.

Most accidents are caused by one or more of four failure levels:

- Organisational influences.
- Unsafe supervision.
- Preconditions for unsafe acts.
- The unsafe acts themselves.

The Threat and Error Management Model

Accidents are rare, but this means that simple accident rates are insensitive statistical measures of safety, making it difficult to assess the effectiveness of different interventions. This limitation was what motivated the development of the University of Texas Threat and Error Management model or TEM (see **Figure 5.3** overpage).

This model classifies the causes of adverse outcomes into threats and errors. Threats are *not* errors – they are the circumstances that provoke them. The term *hazard* is also used in a similar manner. These are examples:

- Ice on the road is a *threat*
—but driving too fast is an *error*.

- Allergy to penicillin is a *threat*
—but giving an allergic person penicillin is an *error*.

- A missing identity bracelet on a patient is a *threat*
—but taking the wrong patient into theatre is an *error*.

The TEM uses three lines of defence against accidents. These are: *avoid*, *trap* and *mitigate*.

AVOID

Much of error avoidance is about recognising threats and—where possible—managing them. With respect to the examples above:

- Ice on the roads can be managed by gritting.
- Hospital notes include prominently displayed warnings about allergy.
- When identity bracelets have to be removed from patients, they should be replaced, on another limb as soon as possible.

TRAP

When errors do occur they do not always lead to disaster. The error can be "trapped" with no adverse consequences. For example:

- A driver can slow down on an icy road.
- The wrong patient can be returned to the ward (and the right one collected).

MITIGATE

The error can have bad consequences that can be mitigated, thus leading to a good outcome. For example:

- Giving penicillin to an allergic patient can be mitigated by treating the patient with adrenaline, steroids and fluid.

An error can lead to a bad outcome because it is not—or cannot be—mitigated. This is illustrated in **Figure 5.2** in which threats and errors are managed by getting to the dotted boxes via the shortest possible route. The longer the route taken, the greater the risk of an adverse outcome and the greater the cost and stress for team members.

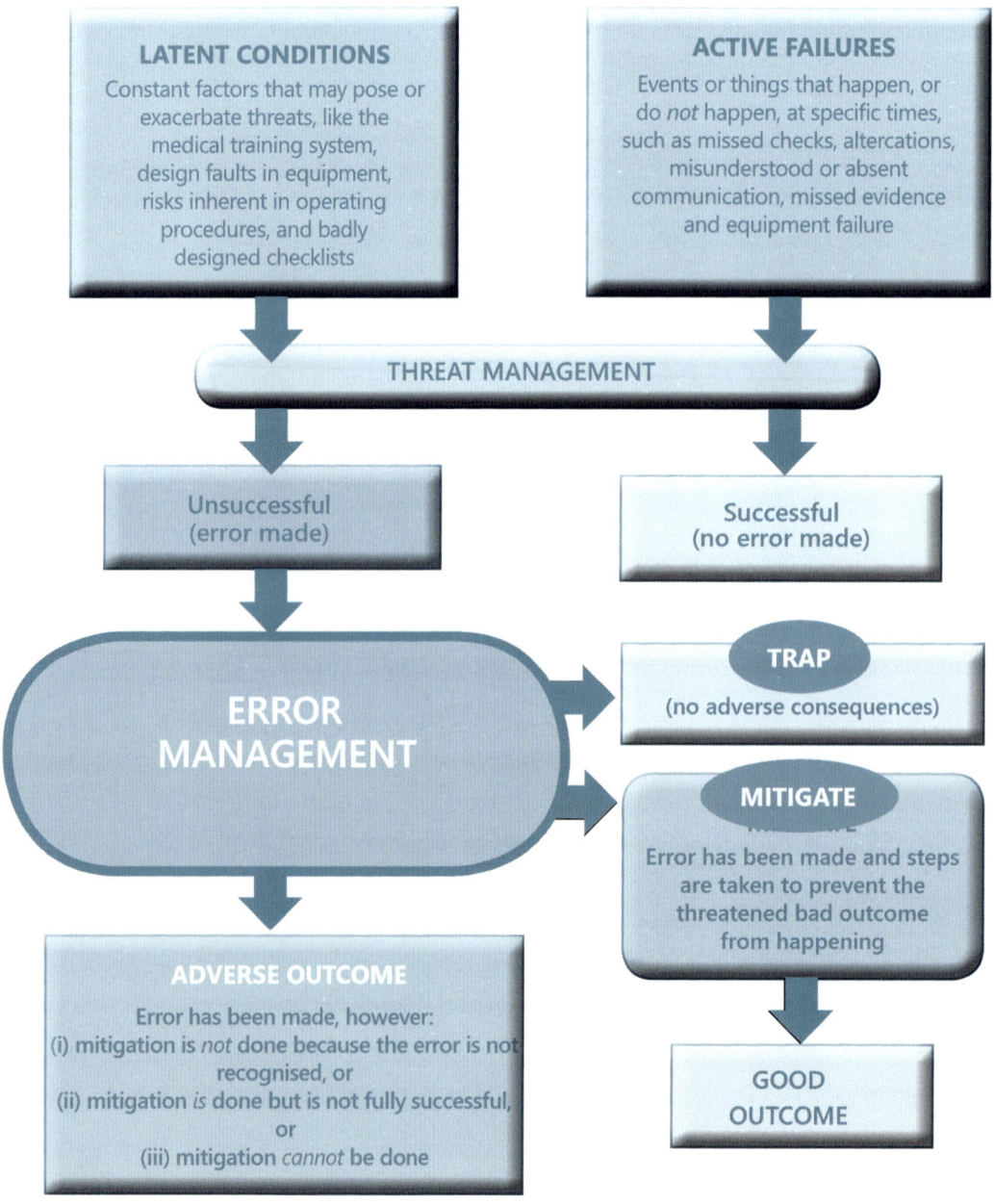

Figure 5.2 *The University of Texas Threat and Error Management (TEM) Model.*

Application of the TEM

The TEM was developed for the aviation industry. Accidents in commercial aviation are caused by series of coincident minor errors and misunderstandings – the so-called "accident chain". These are very common, but accidents are rare.

People investigating accidents only had access to data on a small proportion of such incidents so, in order to reduce accident rates, more data was needed. This led to gathering data outside the context of accidents. Voluntary reporting of near misses is now commonplace in aviation, as is professional observation of cockpit behaviour. Airlines have also adopted real-time monitoring and reporting of aircraft performance as a means of trapping and mitigating errors.

The same applies to healthcare. Mortality rates and quality-of-life measures remain a goal of research, but they are insensitive, and they require large and expensive studies. Surrogate markers are used in the early stages of research; in the case of safety and human factors, threats and errors are those surrogates.

> **Vignette 5.1 Intrathecal vincristine**
>
> Wayne Jowett died in 2001 in a Nottingham hospital. Chemotherapy for his leukaemia comprised two drugs: cytosine (to be given via a lumbar puncture) and vincristine (to be given intravenously).
>
> A registrar supervising a senior house office (SHO) passed the cytosine, then the vincristine. The SHO wrongly administered both to the patient via the lumbar puncture. It was a lethal error.

It occurred despite product warnings, a body of literature that stresses the dangers, previous well-publicised cases and local protocols, in addition to elaborate pharmacy defences that included procedures to ensure that the drugs were never administered at the same time. Numerous background threats and errors conspired to cause the disaster:

- Senior doctors assumed that the juniors knew their subject (it was later argued that the relevant induction and training systems had been faulty)
—a *threat*.

- In the registrar's previous workplace, two syringes containing different drugs were commonly given simultaneously via lumbar puncture
—a *threat*.

- The patient had arrived late for his therapy and extra efforts had been made to accommodate him before the day-ward closed
—a *threat*.

- The staff member who went to collect the drugs from the pharmacy did not know that they should be separated, so they were transported together
—an *error*.

- The nurse who delivered them to the bedside also brought them together
—an *error*.

- The registrar did not notice that the vincristine was to be given intravenously
—an *error*.

- The registrar did not notice that the vincristine was prescribed for the following day
—an *error*.

- The labelling and the general appearance of the two syringes was similar
—a *threat*.

- The registrar said that at one stage he thought the second drug was methotrexate (which is given via lumbar puncture), partly because vincristine should not be available on the same day
—an *error*.

- The SHO was surprised to be given a second syringe and queried the drug and the route verbally, but this was not sufficiently challenging to abort the disaster that followed
—a *failed opportunity to TRAP*.

- Connectors for both the syringes (to either the lumbar puncture needle or to the intravenous cannula) were interchangeable *
—a *threat*.

* Note: this was still the case in 2013 although change was imminent.

The error, therefore, was caused by a long chain of latent conditions that created a threat, and active failures that could have been "trapped". In this scenario, mitigation was not possible.

Conclusions

There is now evidence to show that effective team-work leads to improved patient outcomes, reduces costs, and improves staff morale. Certain elements of human-factors training that has been developed in aviation over the past twenty-five years can be extrapolated to medical teams, provided that the key differences in medicine are recognised.

Leadership

Key points for reflection

❶ Different leadership styles tend to deliver different outcomes for staff and patients.

❷ There are some key features of effective leaders wherever they sit within an organisation.

❸ Different styles of leadership may be needed for different situations, but the effective leader is able to recognise, acknowledge and act upon such contingencies.

The prominent position of leaders has made them a topic of study for centuries. Plato considered that leaders should be taken from the ruling class and specifically educated to lead. They should take personal responsibility for the common good and put this priority over issues such as honesty with the populace. Plato made a distinction between ruling by law and the art of ruling by persuasion.

Machiavelli (1469–1527) discussed fear and love, concepts analogous to Plato's law and persuasion. He noted that leaders should appear to govern virtuously, but in reality act on expediency. They should be seen to be merciful, faithful, humane, frank and religious, but not actually be these things. Machiavelli deals with the issues of generosity versus meanness, honesty versus reputation, and cruelty versus kindness with a similarly expedient rather than principled approach. Most famous is his belief that within certain limits it is better to be feared than to be loved. Five hundred years on, Machiavelli remains one of the most controversial – and widely read – writers on leadership. Widely read, because his advice is seen as effective. Controversial, because it is also seen as immoral!

Nineteenth-century studies on leadership sought personal characteristics or traits that were common among effective leaders. Thomas Carlisle assessed the traits of great historical figures, while Francis Galton studied the leadership skills of the blood relatives of powerful individuals; he found that these skills declined from first-degree to second-degree relationships, and concluded that leadership skills were inherited rather than learned.

This theory of inherited leadership traits (intelligence, morality, self-confidence, adaptability and persistence) was highly influential in psychology in England and indirectly in areas such as education policy. Machiavelli aside, most models remained trait-based and descriptive and did not attempt to instruct on how to lead. Trait theory fails to explain why people who are good leaders in one situation are not necessarily good in another. Improved methods of research led to the idea that both the situation a leader finds him or herself in and their personality traits, are predictive of their performance.

Leadership style

Leadership style is an alternative way of classifying leaders to their traits and situations. Styles refer to their behaviour patterns.

Kurt Lewin (1890–1947) conducted a famous leadership experiment on ten-year-old boys, whom he gave specific group tasks to complete, like making model aeroplanes.

Each group had an adult leader who assumed a different leadership style. Their effect on the individual groups was then compared. Lewin was particularly interested in the effect of leadership style on the boys' levels of aggression.

The experiment was designed to compare democratic and authoritarian (or autocratic) styles, but a "laissez-faire" group was also included as a control to represent "minimum leadership". The styles and definitions he used are shown in **Table 6.1**.

Table 6.1 *Styles and definitions used by leaders in Lewin's experiments*

Authoritarian	Democratic	Laissez-faire
■ Leader determined policy	■ Leader assisted group to determine policies and decisions	■ Leader did not participate in decisions ■ Group had complete freedom over group and individual decisions
■ Leader dictated techniques and steps one at a time ■ Future steps were unknown to a large degree	■ Activity was planned during the first discussion period with general steps sketched out ■ Leader suggested two or three alternatives from which the group chose, when technical advice was needed	■ Leader supplied materials and made it clear that information would be supplied when asked for ■ Leader took no other part in discussions
■ Leader dictated who did what task and who worked in which subgroup	■ Group members were free to work with whoever they chose ■ Whole group decided how tasks were divided	■ Leader did not participate
■ Leader was friendly or impersonal, but not openly hostile and did not participate in activities except to demonstrate	■ Leader was objective with both praise and criticism and tried to be a regular group member in spirit without doing too much of the work	■ Leader made infrequent comments on member's activities unless questioned ■ Leader made no attempt to participate or interfere with the course of events

Lewin's main findings were.

- **Aggression** between the boys was eight times greater in the authoritarian group than in the democratic group. The boys' reaction to the authoritarian leader involved submission or attention seeking. In two cases, the generalised inter-member aggression condensed into aggression against an individual boy. In both situations, the boys left the experiment, and in both cases the leader saw the "victims" as natural group leaders.

- **Egocentric behaviour** occurred twice as much in the authoritarian group than the democratic group.

Later experiments suggested two things:

> ■ Groups that are under stress perform better under authoritarian leadership.
>
> ■ Groups that are not under stress are more productive and better quality when under democratic leadership.

Authoritarian leadership is at its *best* when the team members are under stress and the leader's judgement and decision-making is the best in the group. If a leader has greater seniority, experience and knowledge than their team, this does not alone imply that an authoritarian style is best. It is at its *worst* when a leader lacks direct experience of the front-line tasks of the team, and lacks the intelligence to recognise their own limitations.

Democratic leadership is at its *best* under relatively low-stress situations and if there are complex tasks, particularly if these require a number of people working in different specialist areas. In such situations, the leader is not likely to have detailed knowledge of each person's specialty. They do not need detailed knowledge of any of the specialties if their democratic leadership skills are good. The widespread success of the democratic leadership style means that people with these skills tend to do well wherever they are. It is at its *worst* in high-stress situations, with inexperienced teams and a leader who is experienced in all aspects of the team's task (the same situation in which authoritarian leadership is at its best).

The basic styles in Lewin's experiments, and their associated group performances, have been repeatedly confirmed in other experiments. The "laissez-faire" style has been treated as an actual style rather than just a control group, as was intended, and other styles have been added, including "toxic" styles. Lewin's democratic and authoritarian styles have been developed into theories of situational leadership whereby leaders adapt their styles to suit their situation.

Situational models

Leadership style theories make group performance a function of the leader's style and the situation. Situational leadership theories make style a variable as well. Good leaders can suite many situations by adapting themselves to them. Lewin's styles of authoritarian, democratic and laissez-faire have been suggested to suit situations of urgent crisis, day-to-day management and creative problem-solving, respectively. The best known situational leadership model is the Hersey–Blanchard Model.

The Hersey–Blanchard Model

This model proposes four leadership styles based on two behavioural domains – task-driven and relationship-driven (**Table 6.2**).

Table 6.2 *Matrix of Hersey–Blanchard leadership styles*

Relationship driven	Task driven	
	HIGH	LOW
HIGH	**S2: Selling** — The leader gives direction, social and emotional support using two-way communication to influence rather than dictate	**S3: Participating** — Prioritises group friendship and cooperation above completion of the task, and shares decision making with group members
LOW	**S1: Telling** — The leader decides what to do and how to do it and tells the group in one-way communication	**S4: Delegating** — Involved in direction, but mainly by monitoring, handing responsibility for process details to individuals or the group

The other central part of their model is a system of classifying followers into four levels of maturity derived from two domains – competence and commitment.

People have different levels of maturity for different tasks, so someone who is level M4 for their job may be M1 if asked to do something they think is not worth bothering with (**Table 6.3**).

Table 6.3 *Hersey–Blanchard levels of maturity among followers*

Level	Characteristics
M1	Incompetent or unwilling to do the task or take responsibility it
M2	Not competent, but are willing to gain the necessary competence and do the task
M3	Competent to do the task, but are not aware of this and think that they are not
M4	Can do the task, know they can do it and are willing to do it

Effective leadership depends on matching the leadership style to both the task and the follower maturity. A good leader's behaviour is then a function of the followers they are dealing with, as well as their personality and the situation.

The Transactional/Transformational Model

Eric Berne developed the idea of transactional analysis in which interpersonal dealings are seen as transactions along the lines of:

> *"I get what I want from you in exchange for giving you what you want."*

Applying this idea to the relationship between leaders and followers led to the concept of *transactional leadership*.

- A *transactional* leader has external reward or coercive power and their team follows them in exchange for reward or avoidance of punishment. Transactional leaders work on the rational conscious level of their followers.

- A *transformational* leader, on the other hand, does not engage in deal-making to get a job done but motivates followers emotionally. They are visible, good communicators, conscious of the ultimate aims of what the group is doing, and use non-power based methods to achieve them.

The differences between them are shown in **Table 6.4**.

Table 6.4 *Differences between transformational and transactional leaders*

Transactional leadership	Transformational leadership
■ Head down	■ Head up
■ Focuses on the practical	■ Focuses on the possible
■ Coaches/directs	■ Inspires
■ Does the job right	■ Does the right job
■ Harnesses or directs energy	■ Creates energy
■ Turns ideas into reality	■ Has vision and ideas
■ Focuses on the next intermediate objective	■ Focuses on ultimate objectives
■ Performance oriented	■ People oriented
■ Sets objectives	■ Questions assumptions
■ Fixes problems	■ Creates problems

Toxic leaders

A toxic leader is one who leaves a group or organisation worse off than they found it. The usual reason is a failure to match their style to the situation. The most common type of toxic leader is the inflexible autocrat. The mistakes they make are:

- **Poor decision making**—They do not see that other group members have a better view of what to do than themselves, so they do not seek group input.

- **Capriciousness**—Consultation and agreement tends to lead to moderate, stable decisions that are neither brilliant nor disastrous. Autocratic decisions are more liable to be brilliant or disastrous – disastrous in incompetent hands of course, but less stable, and prone to sudden unexpected reversal.

- **Alienation of the group**—Team members who do not feel dependent on the leader and are never consulted or involved in policy, quickly lose interest.

- **Frequent aggression**—Lewin's original observation was of a higher rate of inter-member aggression within autocratically led groups than within democratically led groups.

Toxic democratic leaders are rare. In situations where they have the knowledge and experience to determine what to do – and those around them do not – they still dither and ask for further input into decision-making. One thing that saves democratic leaders in this situation is that they can recognise which of their group members are able to take on an autocratic role when needed, and can use them to coordinate the required autocratic component of leadership while themselves maintaining group cohesion and motivation with a democratic style.

Apparatchik

A common version of the toxic autocrat is the *apparatchik* (from the Russian description of middle-ranking Communist Party officials). Apparatchiks accept without question what their superiors ask of them, then they brook no opposition from inferiors when carrying out these orders. They work to rules and are poor at taking personal responsibility.

When no rule can be found to address a problem, they ask those above them what to do. Consequently they appear as compliant, but needy and unimaginative functionaries to their superiors, and as inflexible pedantic autocrats to their inferiors.

They are common in situations where middle-ranking managers are appointed by their superiors and in large rigidly bureaucratic organisations, where such behaviour is frequently rewarded. Working under an apparatchik is no fun, but their real danger to an organisation is in converting the two-way discourse between frontline staff and senior management into a one-way autocratic communication channel.

Inverse apparatchik

The inverse apparatchik is unshakably cynical about people above them in the command structure, believing them to be incompetent, self-serving and corrupt. They see themselves – and those below them – as dutiful, competent and exploited, and they vigorously defend the interests of their colleagues and subordinates or patients. They are common in situations where middle-ranking managers are elected by their peers or juniors. The problem is that they cannot – or will not – see issues from the strategic, expedient point of view. When they succeed in their parochial aims, they can seriously undermine – or even ruin – the organisation.

Command structure in healthcare

The above models were based on people appointed to roles of leadership in organisations that use a single pyramidal command structure such as fire-fighting organisations, the police force and the military. At each level of the pyramid there is a leader who is in charge of usually between two and ten individuals. This structure is often reinforced by visible symbols. This kind of command structure is referred to by Henry Mintzberg as a "machine-like".

In healthcare, such appointed leaders are not so apparent. The UK's NHS has at least three command pyramids: doctors, nursing and administration. In a team such as that of an operating theatre, different members are answerable to different command lines rather than to a single team leader. Nurses are answerable to the nursing hierarchy, administrative staff to their own hierarchy, and doctors to consultants. The doctors have a command pyramid of medical directors, clinical directors, heads of departments, consultants and juniors, but the rankings above consultant do not apply to the operational front-line; this gives a flat command structure with large numbers of consultants who are independent practitioners of equivalent seniority. This is what Mintzberg describes as a "professional bureaucracy".

A PROFESSIONAL BUREAUCRACY HAS THESE PREDICTED PROPERTIES—

- Stability is prioritised over change.
- Work is organised in many multidisciplinary groups.
- The function of leadership is distributed to many professionals.
- Leadership skills training is important for many groups.

THE FRONT-LINE STAFF HAVE—

- Control over work content.
- More influence than appointed managers on day-to-day decisions.

THE LEADERS HAVE TO NEGOTIATE CHANGES RATHER THAN IMPOSE THEM

- Hierarchical directives have little effect.
- Positional power is not always followed or respected.
- Influence is more significant in achieving change.
- Professional networks and peer pressure are important.
- Professional credibility is important.

The result is that large numbers of NHS employees need particularly democratic leadership skills.

Leadership and power

- *Power* is the ability to threaten punishment or offer reward.
- *Leadership* is the ability to bring a group of people to effective action.

With professional bureaucracies, who has power for front-line operations is often ambiguous, and consequently recourse to power can lead to conflict; even if it is clear who has power, it is often more effective for them not to exercise it overtly.

We draw a distinction between leadership with and without the exercise of power. Not everyone has a job in which they can exercise power, but leadership can be exercised in many ways, depending on a person's skills, making leadership training relevant to everyone.

- **Leadership is *more effective* than power—**
Power can take a horse to water but it cannot make it drink; leadership takes a horse to water when it is thirsty.

- **Leadership is *better* than power—**
If something needs to be done, it will be done better, faster and more efficiently if it is coordinated by leadership than if it is coordinated by power.

Only when leadership fails is it necessary to resort to power, and the frequency with which people do resort to power is inversely proportional to their leadership skill.

Credibility

Credibility is that quality in a leader that means that their team members respect their opinions. It is something that others observe in the leader; the leader has little direct short-term control over it. It is based on consistency of behaviour over weeks and months.

Credibility and personality type

People view the credibility of others according their own personality type:

- Guardians are inclined to assume that people in authority must be credible. They tend to respect reliability, serious-mindedness and worthy objectives.
- Artisans give credibility to people with grace and taste.
- Idealists give credibility not so much to effectiveness but to creditable motivations.
- Rationals do not accept the credibility of leaders because of their position, but only because of their grasp and usage of reasoned explanations for their actions.

Similarly, Feeling people find sensitivity credible, whereas Thinking people find logic credible.

> **The best leaders change their approach according to who they are dealing with, and will appear:**
>
> ■ *Logical* to Rationals
>
> ■ *Tasteful* to Artisans
>
> ■ *Responsible* to Guardians
>
> ■ *Empathetic* to Idealists
>
> This skill is learned from experience and comes to be acted on automatically—it is not taught.

Credibility and intelligence (IQ)

The credibility of leaders increases with intelligence and education, and falls with increasing levels of intelligence and education among their followers. In healthcare many professionals have high levels of education. It can be difficult to appear credible to doctors without equivalent qualifications. It also means that the consultant bodies of healthcare organisations are among the most difficult to lead and influence.

Emotional intelligence

Leadership is an emotion-laden activity and several attempts have been made to model and measure people's performance with emotional issues.

Daniel Goleman defined the Emotional Intelligence Quota (EQ) of five domains:

- Knowing one's own emotions.
- Managing one's own emotions.
- Self-motivation.
- Understanding other people's emotions.
- Managing relationships.

He found that EQ correlated better with success than the intelligence quotient (IQ).

The Emotional and Social Competency Inventory (ESCI) and the Emotional Intelligence Appraisal are derived from Goleman's model. Salovey and Mayer's Ability Model is based on ability to perceive, use, understand and manage emotions and is behind the Mayer–Salovey–Caruso Emotional Intelligence Test (MSCEIT).

K.V. Petrides developed an EI model based on observed characteristics rather than skills or abilities, and measures have been derived from it including the EQ-i, the Swinburne University Emotional Intelligence Test (SUEIT) and Trait Emotional Intelligence Questionnaire (TEIQue). However, some question whether EI is really a distinct psychological entity – as opposed to another way of expressing personality traits – and question its value in prediciting career success.

Training leadership

Leadership skills can be taught in a two-phase process:

- **Phase 1**—Learning concepts and tools of leadership.
- **Phase 2**— Practical experience with changing situations and individuals, which is maximised by honest and respectful feedback from other people.

Here are some of the tools of effective leadership.

1. SHOW, DON'T TELL

Increasing education, especially in softer sciences, makes people increasingly sceptical about the conclusions of others. The more sophisticated audiences become, the more leaders or instructors should show evidence and allow them to draw their own conclusions rather than drawing conclusions and expecting them to be accepted in the absence of the evidence. Medical personnel rarely tell each other what to do; they ask for advice, they present evidence, and they discuss the implications of that evidence.

2. LEADING BY EXAMPLE

People with credible leadership are closely watched and copied by those around them. Good leaders know this and choose to do things in a way that is easy and safe to copy, rather than glamorous or flashy. Actions speak louder than words.

3. MOTIVATION

Motivation and credibility are linked – people are poorly motivated to work with a team leader who lacks credibility, but motivation is easier to teach. Points 4-8 below promote motivation.

4. POSITIVE REINFORCEMENT

Positive reinforcement means responding to something another person does in a way that encourages them to do it again, generally by appreciating, thanking or praising them. For example, take a surgeon who occasionally holds a pre-list briefing; if, on those occasions, the other theatre staff thank him and say how the briefing helped the list run much more smoothly, then the surgeon is more likely to carry out such briefings more often.

5. BUY-IN

Team members should feel possession of the process. When a team member has an idea, they should be identified with it; this will encourage them to make it succeed. When the leader's idea has input from other team members, the leader should let them feel the idea is theirs.

6. USE OF BLAME

Just as crediting team members with success draws them to the leader and motivates them to perform, blaming them for failures drives them away and demotivates them. There are occasions when blame is either obvious or could be apportioned. The motivational approach is to separate the problems and issues from the people. Even if someone is clearly to blame, it is more likely to be due to their lack of training, poor team communication, or inappropriate personnel deployment than deliberate sabotage.

7. DELEGATION OF TASKS

The default position of task delegation in teams is for the same tasks to be given to the same people time and time again. These tasks are distributed from the most important or interesting to senior members, to the most straightforward, repetitive and dull to junior members. Changing this pattern of delegation can be highly motivational. Giving more junior team members tasks they are capable of, but do not generally get (and may not know they can do), both develops and motivates them.

8. COMMONALITY OF PURPOSE

Commonality of purpose requires that all the people involved in a project agree with its methods and ultimate goals. Achieving commonality requires leaders to see the situation from different points of view: their own, the team members', the patients' and the organisation as a whole.

Conflicts between the interests of the team and the organisation do arise and require balanced judgement and background explanations to resolve. From a balanced understanding of the needs of all involved, commonality of purpose is gained when the leader communicates to explain the aims, and is sufficiently flexible to change any proposals and methods of achieving them to concur with those of others.

9. TEAM MEMBER DEVELOPMENT

Very few leaders attract a significant following that endures long after their death. Those few that have achieved this, such as the founders of the world's great religions, were characterised by their tendency to prioritise the development of others over their own interests. Developing other team members is the way in which leaders secure the most lasting loyalty and respect.

10. VISIBILITY

Visible leaders are easy to find and approach. They have offices that are located conveniently and they spend time in and around the teams they lead. Visibility is limited by time constraints and there is a need for balance, but there is no more effective way of achieving one's own objectives than by motivating others to share them and work towards them too.

11. HUMOUR

All organisations contain serious-minded people who tend to look down on humour as a frivolous and distracting waste of time. The conclusion of the research on this matter is the opposite. Data from a range of working environments show that appropriate use of humour can improve productivity, team-work, morale and work-related stress. It can defuse anger and soften reprimands. It allows things to be said that would be unacceptable in a serious context. It can help with problem-solving, decision-making, and enhancing creativity. The main disadvantage is that humorous statements can be turned against the maker by opponents. Humour can also be viewed as a way of trivialising issues, or being denigrating, flippant or prejudiced. That is why official documents, protocols, manifestoes, and the like never contain humour.

12. DIFFUSION OF RESPONSIBILITY

Diffusion of responsibility refers to a tendency for people to take less responsibility for their actions (or inactions) when others are present because they assume others will take necessary actions. It is prone to occur in groups of three or more people and is more likely to happen if tasks and responsibilities have not been specifically assigned. It is a risk of the democratic leadership style; the solution is for clear allocation of responsibility. The authoritarian style is also affected by diffusion of responsibility; subordinates readily disengage themselves from everything except what they have been instructed to do, and do not make allowances for changing situations without new instructions. When adverse events occur, subordinates later claim to have been "just following orders" while supervisors claim their role was to "give instructions – not carry them out". Such explanations have followed many crimes against humanity; the solution is more democratic engagement of group members.

Medical Leadership Competency Framework (MLCF)

The MLCF is an NHS leadership training program aimed at doctors. Dating from 2008, it was developed by the NHS Institute for Innovation and Improvement and the Academy of Medical Royal Colleges. It has since been adopted by other NHS policy documents and is intended to be taught to medical students, doctors in training, consultants and GPs. The MLCF uses one model of leadership, referred to as shared leadership. In this model, any doctor can perform acts of leadership whether or not they hold a designated leadership role. It contains no discussion on leadership styles, but the style it promotes is strongly democratic. It is structured into five main themes covering personal qualities, working with others, managing service, improving services, and setting directions. The attributes it confers on effective leaders in the NHS are shown in **Figure 6.1** overpage.

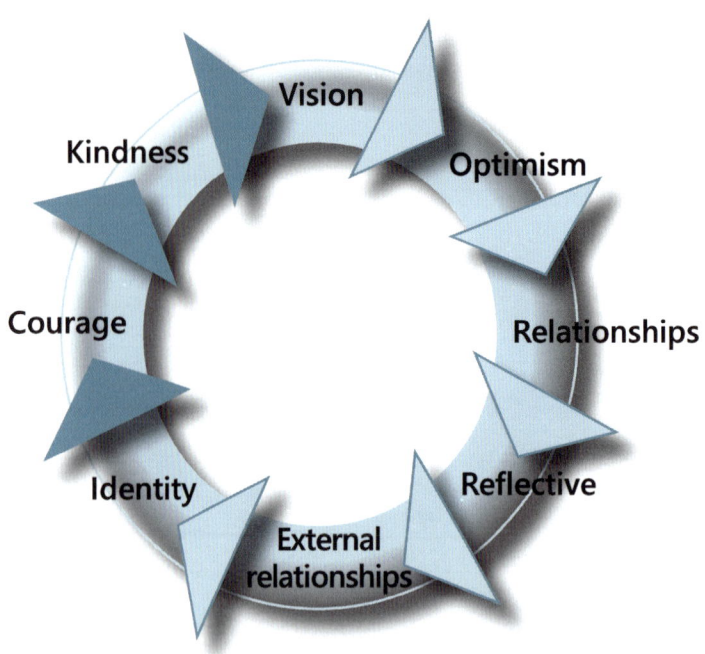

Figure 6.1 *Key attributes of effective leaders in the NHS.*

Strengths and weakness of the MLCF

Its *strengths* are that it has been officially incorporated into undergraduate, postgraduate and continuing medical education in the UK. It is also clear and specific.

Its *weaknesses* are that its teaching style is autocratic: it does not show, it tells; it cites no evidence and it invites no debate. Furthermore, it includes issues that are more about policies that were current at the time it was written (such as systems of appraisal, reflective practice and multidisciplinary team meetings) than about leadership.

Conclusions

The two basic styles of leadership are *democratic* and *authoritarian*. Both have their strengths and weaknesses and suit different situations. The best leaders adopt a "situational approach" whereby their leadership style is adapted to suite the situation. Western societies in general (and healthcare in particular) have evolved over the last few generations from a primarily autocratic leadership style to a primarily democratic style that better suits the complex, multidisciplinary demands of modern clinical practice.

Communication

Key points for reflection

❶ Communications often benefit from particular structuring, depending on the situation.

❷ Both 'sender' and 'receiver' characteristics are important in understanding effective communications.

❸ Do not be afraid to give colleagues a "good listening to".

Communication failures are common contributors to medical mishaps. Serious adverse events (SAE) occur in 5–20% of NHS patients, incurring high costs on the NHS (for example, costs were estimated at two billion pounds in 2003). Communication errors contribute to as much as 80% of cases. In the USA, data indicate that in over 75% of sentinel events in healthcare, poor communication is among the root causes.

Without thought or training, people tend to act on impulse with simple reactions that focus on short-term self-interests. The alternative to impulse is reflection which requires consideration, thought or training, without which impulse remains the default. Tasks that are particularly prone to impulsive behaviour are those that require little concentration or thought. First amongst these is speaking in one's mother tongue, which is why impulse versus reflection is such an issue in communication. Various aspects of communication skills are described below. If there is one over-riding message for improving our communication, it is:

"Think before speaking!"

Communication theory

In 1949, Shannon and Weaver of the Bell telephone laboratory divided communication into the phases of encoding, transmission and decoding of the message. Any message is subject to noise (interference) during transmission. This model was expanded by Berlo into four parts, creating the SMCR model. Where S stands for Sender, M stands for Message, C stands for Channel, and R stands for Receiver.

All parts of this process are subject to noise, and errors arising at any stage are transmitted through the rest of the stages, so the final error rate is cumulative (see **Figure 7.1** overpage).

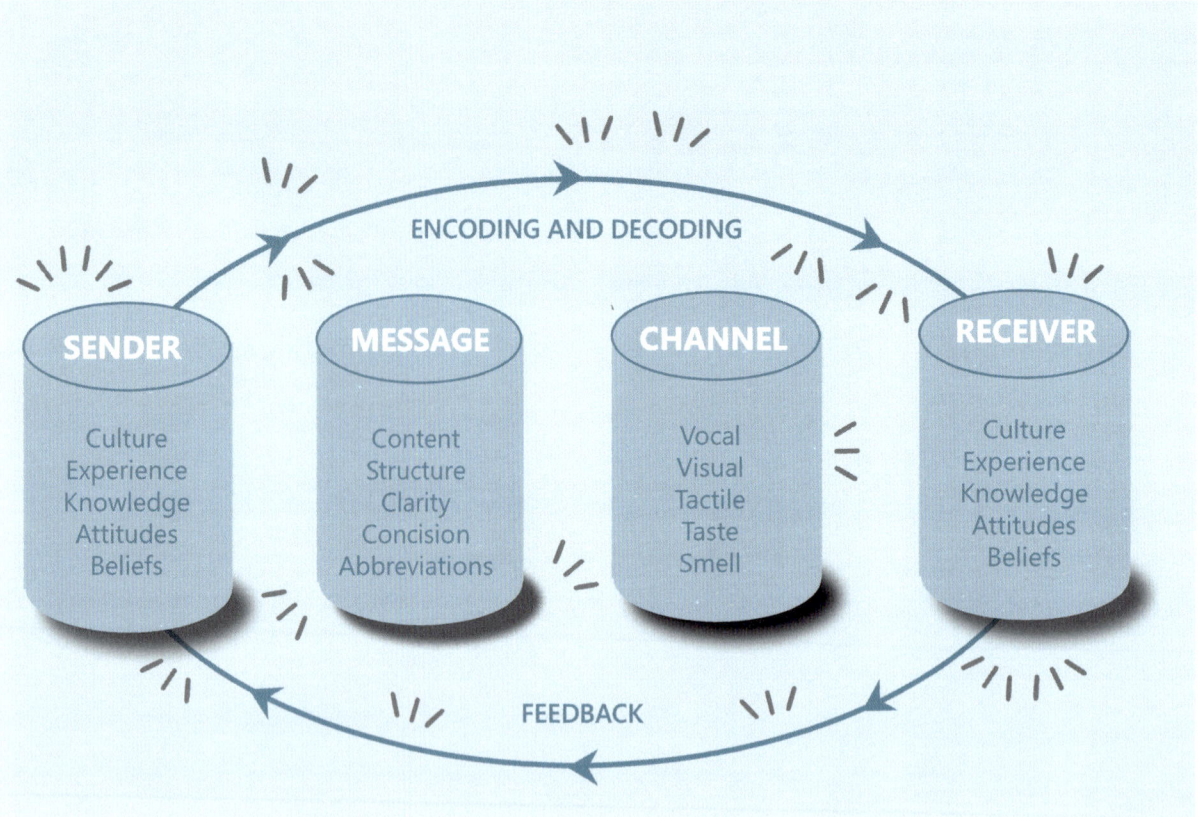

Figure 7.1 *Sender–Message–Channel–Receiver (SMCR) communication model with feedback.*

The importance of feedback in communication was addressed by Schramm in 1954. In this model, communication goes from the Sender to the Receiver and back again. This feedback can either confirm that the receiver has understood what the sender intended, or it can be corrective.

Sender (SMCR)

The sender is the speaker or writer of a message. According to Robert Bolton, a sender can have three characteristics that enhance the effectiveness of their communication – whatever the message might be:

- Genuineness (without false front or façade)
- Respect (patience, fairness, consistency, rationality, kindliness towards another)
- Empathy (understanding of another person's perspective)

And according to Thomas Gordon there are twelve "roadblocks" within the three groups that make a sender less effective – whatever the message:

GROUP I—Judging the other person rather than focusing on the issue

- Criticising
- Giving abuse
- Diagnosing the sender's "hidden agenda"
- Evaluative praising

Module Seven: Communication

GROUP II—Sending solutions rather than agreeing them

- Ordering
- Threatening
- Moralising
- Using leading questions
- Advising

GROUP III—Ignoring the receiver's concerns and input

- Diverting
- Logical argument
- Reassuring

The second two of Gordon's groups are "roadblocks" but they have a quick impact, and in a crisis they may be the only options. The best level of assertiveness is a balanced judgment. It can be escalated in stages, such as those outlined in the PACE (Probe–Alert–Challenge–Emergency) sequence described in *Module 3*.

Message (sMcr)

The tone of the message is important, and for *dispassionate* communication, it should be clear, short and focused on the issue at hand – not on the Sender or Receiver. This approach frequently conflicts with emotional communication so it is not always appropriate.

To tell a patient that "*You have cancer, and with the best treatment available the prognosis of your condition is a median survival time of twelve months…*" is generally not good communication. Clarity and accuracy often have to be balanced against empathy.

Much of the subtlety we put into communication for emotional reasons does not translate well into other cultures or languages and is liable to lead to confusion. When speaking to someone with a limited grasp of English, softening a blow by saying "*I would rather not*" instead of "*I will not*" is liable to lead to a misunderstanding.

The size of the message is also important. On average only five pieces of information can be kept in a person's short-term memory. The Receiver can be overload by more than five pieces of information in one message, or if too many messages are sent at the same time. If numerous points or messages are necessary, then the Sender can help the Receiver by providing a written copy of the message and by making the relative priority of the different points clear. Messages come in two basic types: mechanistic and transformational.

MECHANISTIC AND TRANSFORMATIONAL MESSAGES.

Mechanistic messages are like those of a machine. They are simple facts that can be passed from one person to another in a stream, like dates of birth, blood pressures and drug doses. There is no need for the person handling the message to understand its meaning. Transformational messages send understanding of systems or emotional feelings to the Receiver. They are so called because they change, or transform, both the Receiver's and the Sender's mental models. Of the two types, *transformational* messages are the more demanding to communicate accurately.

STRUCTURED MESSAGES

Structured messages use a formula to present pieces of information in a pre-agreed order, designed to avoid missing important things. In medicine there is a pre-agreed structure for case histories (patient age and sex, presentation, history of the presenting complaint, previous medical history, examination findings, investigation results and treatment plan). Structured communication is illustrated in **Figure 7.2**. The structured message makes it much easier to spot when something missing. Structured messages are good for mechanistic messages, but poor for transformational messages. Purely structured communication ignores the associations between items and imposes a list-type structure to ensure that nothing is missed out.

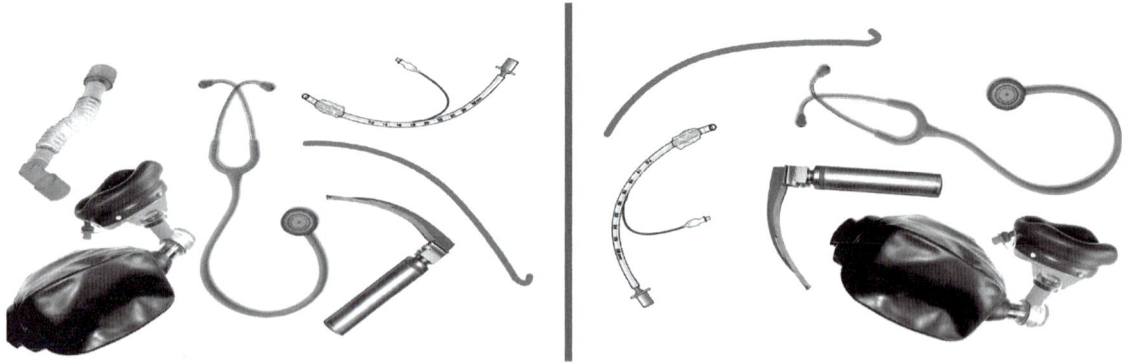

Figure 7.2a *The left-hand panel shows all the equipment needed for intubation. In the right-hand panel, one item is missing. It takes time to spot which one, and without knowing that something is missing, it may go unnoticed.*

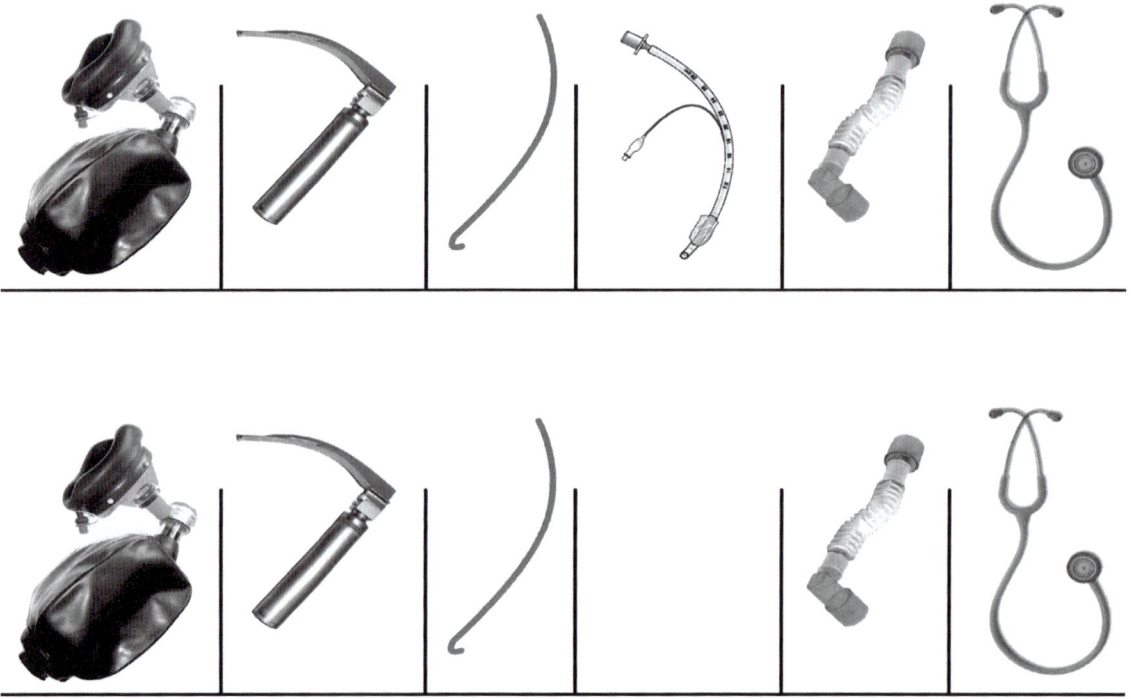

Figure 7.2b *The same equipment, but presented in a structured fashion. In the lower panel one thing is missing, but now it is easy to spot it, and without knowing that something was missing, it would still be noticeable.*

NARRATIVE MESSAGES

In narrative, or "storytelling" messages, the items communicated all either state or support a common premise, based on the associations between items. Narrative communication is much easier to understand than structured communication, and it is the best method for transformational communication. The narrative approach starts with the most important facts to communicate and then fills in the background as supporting information. Producing a good narrative takes careful forethought. When you have a message to send that suits narrative, preview what you plan to say before saying it. Ask:

- What is the main point?
- Could it be shortened?
- Could it be clarified?
- Are there things that do not add to the message I could omit?
- Are there things that do add to the message that I could include?
- Have I got the main point first and supporting information second?
- Is the supporting information organised for maximum clarity?

STRUCTURED–NARRATIVE MESSAGES

There have been various attempts to combine narrative and structured messages. The best known tool is SBAR, which is recommended by the UK Resuscitation Council Guidelines 2010. SBAR stands for:

> **S** ituation
> **B** ackground
> **A** ssessment
> **R** ecommendation

Other structured narrative systems include Five-Step Advocacy, which specifies the use of the Receiver's name (so that the Sender gets the attention of the Receiver) and seeks feedback:

- Step 1—Attention getting (e.g. "*Excuse me, Doctor Lamb*")
- Step 2—Stating a concern (e.g. "*Mr Jones, oxygen saturations are dropping*")
- Step 3—Stating the problem as seen (e.g. "*I think his pneumonia is progressing*")
- Step 4—Stating a solution (e.g. "*Let's give oxygen and contact outreach*")
- Step 5—Obtaining agreement (e.g. "*Does that sound reasonable, Doctor Lamb?*")

These tools are, in essence, structures and they do not help with true narrative communication, which is improved by knowledge, experience and intelligence, all of which are not under our short-term control. What we can do is think before sending.

NARRATIVE VERSUS STRUCTURED MESSAGES

Structured communication helps to prevent the omission of essential things, but it gives little guidance on how to organise a message for ease of comprehension. A narrative approach, on the other hand, allows concepts to be communicated clearly. In **Vignette 7.1** overpage, the same facts are expressed structured and narrative for comparison.

> ### Vignette 7.1   Same message—Two versions
>
> #### Structured message
>
> Surgical registrar calls anaesthetist: *"I am phoning about: Patient—76-year-old man. Complaining of—pain in the back radiating into the right groin. History of presenting complaint—it came on three hours ago and has worsened since. Previous medical history—angina, stable, controlled on nitrates, he can climb one flight of stairs before stopping. Social history—lives with his wife who is fit, smokes twenty cigarettes per day, social drinker. On examination —cold sweat, pulse 100, BP 105/55, tender mass in abdomen? Pulsatile. Vital signs improving with resuscitation. Investigations—CT shows a ruptured abdominal aortic aneurysm below the renal arteries with aneurysmal dilation extending into the left common iliac artery. Plan—urgent transperitoneal repair."*
>
> #### Narrative message
>
> Surgical registrar calls anaesthetist: *"I have a man with a ruptured aortic aneurysm that needs urgent repair. Pulse is currently 100 with BP 105/55 improving with resuscitation. The diagnosis has been confirmed on CT. He is 76 with stable angina, can climb a flight of stairs without stopping and smokes twenty cigarettes per day."*
>
> Surgical registrar rings consultant surgeon: *"We have admitted a 76-year-old man with a ruptured aortic aneurysm. CT shows it to be below the renal arteries but there is aneurysmal dilation of the left common iliac. He's a smoker with a history of stable angina but is otherwise reasonably well. He was in hypovolaemic shock on arrival but is responding to resuscitation."*

The structured version is fine for facts written on a page whereby the reader can skip from place to place. The narrative version is more suited to the serial nature of speech.

Good narrative communication differs from structured communication in two major respects:

- *The speaker organises the points that need to be communicated into a hierarchy of importance* and presents the most important, or essential, features first, followed by the supporting information.

- *The speaker prioritises the information according to what the listener is likely to be interested in* and selects what information to present, depending on who is being spoken to (for example, the anaesthetist in **Vignette 7.1** is interested in the patient's exercise tolerance and smoking habit and less so in the anatomy of the aneurysm, while the consultant surgeon is interested in the technical aspects of the aneurysm and its repair).

In order to form a narrative, the Sender must know the importance of an aneurysm and how it is relates to the patient's clinical condition, the necessary treatment, and what the priorities are from the point of view of the various people being spoken to. This knowledge of associations takes training and experience to acquire.

Narrative communication is at its best when used by experienced members of the team. Less experienced team members may not have the knowledge to use narrative communication effectively and they will depend more on structured communication.

Narrative requires transformational communication. The sender must have a mental model in order to form a narrative. If Jane explains a situation to Peter and Peter then explains it to Tom, Peter cannot simply repeat the Jane's words. He must have understood what Jane said and then form his own narrative. If Peter does not fully understand Jane, his narrative will be inaccurate or incomplete. Structured communication can be passed on from person to person with less reliance on each individual's understanding.

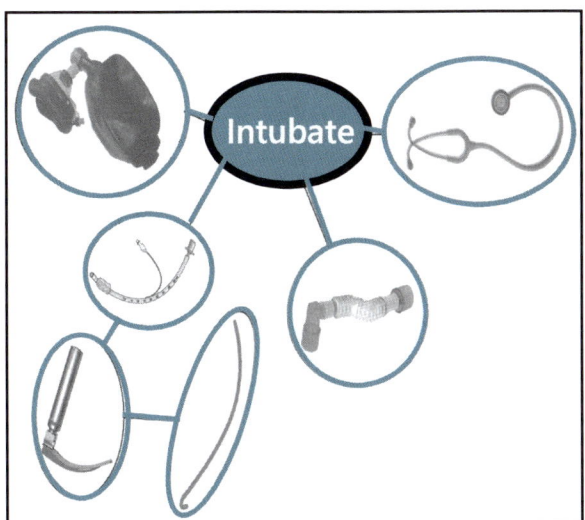 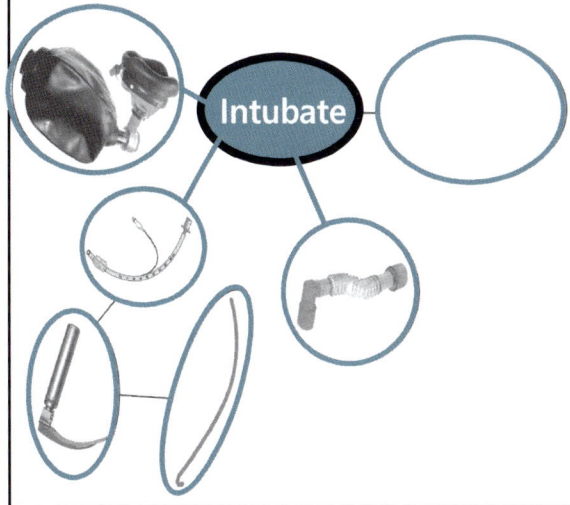

Figure 7.3 *Narrative version of Figures 7.2a and 7.2b. There is something missing. To anyone who is familiar with what is needed to intubate the images flow well and it will be obvious that the stethoscope is missing, but someone who is not familiar with intubation will probably miss it.*

SOUND BITES

A sound bite is a simple, apparently logical or self-evident piece of information that is easily transmitted and remembered. Sound bites pervade communication with multiple people. They are useful for getting a message across, but bias complex issues towards one simple view or another, without any justification. When a message contains a sound bite, it is likely that only the sound bite will be transmitted to most Receivers; none of the supporting information will get through. If there is a sound bite to be communicated, it must be the *right* one. If what is to be communicated is not a sound bite, then no sound bites should be used because they will obscure the message.

A common, special case of the sound bite is the *blame bite*. In **Vignette 7.2**, the heading is the blame bite and is a misleading distortion of the message.

> **Vignette 7.2** Sound bite *"MAN DIES AFTER DRUG ERROR!"*
>
> A man with end-stage emphysema was admitted with a chest infection. Antibiotic treatment was started but the patient worsened and became semiconscious. After discussion between the medical team and family, it was decided that there was no prospect of recovery and the object of treatment should be changed from treating the infection to relieving suffering.
>
> The antibiotics were stopped but the next day one dose was given in error. It made no difference to the situation and the man died peacefully, as expected, a few hours later.

Sound bites form *the* communication link between teams and the world outside. Senior team members are likely to be more sensitive to the consequences of sound bites than more junior members, and this can be divisive because it makes some members appear political, disingenuous and self-serving and thus can lead to acrimony unless the role of sound bites in communication is understood.

COMMUNICATING EMOTION

Rational thought occurs in language. Emotions are felt. The words we communicate with predominantly convey a rational message. Both the tone of the voice and the body language used contribute more significantly to the emotional component.

This is a divide that is surprisingly difficult to cross. It takes considerable skill for a communicator to invoke emotion effectively purely with language, and the expression of rational argument in feelings is extremely difficult. In our minds, however, the link between emotion and reason is intimate.

> Our rational thought tends to follow where positive emotion leads and steers away from negative emotion.

Knowledge of this link assists in effective communication because it can be used for feedback control. We can read people's emotions from their body language and tone, and pursue areas of communication where they are responding favourably. When they are not, we can revise our strategy or content accordingly.

Channel (smCr)

The channel refers to the modalities by which information is exchanged. They include spoken words, tone of voice, facial expressions, gestures and body language, written text and graphic aids.

Non-verbal cues can enhance understanding by:

- Confirming what is being said.
- Contradicting what is being said.
- Emotionally qualifying what is being said.
- Prioritising spoken points.
- Substituting for words.

The relative importance of these factors was investigated in a widely quoted (and misquoted!) series of experiments by Mehrabian and colleagues. They studied words, tone of voice and non-verbal cues that did not agree with each other. When non-verbal cues or tone of voice did not match the words used, they found that: only 7% of the conveyed meaning came from the words; 38% from the tone of voice; and 55% from non-verbal cues.

> The importance of non-verbal cues in communicating the emotional aspects of mental models is widely recognised, but they are equally important in rational models.

The following scenario **(Vignette 7.3)** describes a student's account of learning a highly rational system.

> **Vignette 7.3 Channels of communication**
>
> I took UK's Open University course in quantum mechanics. The teaching material was text books, audio and video programs. There were tutorial group meetings every two weeks but I was not able to attend many because of the shifts I worked.
>
> I applied myself but three months into the course I was lost. I spent hours poring over the course modules, other text books, television programs and popular science books, but could not get my head round the basics of the quantum model. I managed to scrape through the assignments by adapting analogous worked examples – not by real understanding. I thought I was going to fail.
>
> Six months into the course I attended the a one-week summer school. The first evening was encouraging in a way; the other students were just as baffled as I was! We met one of the seasoned tutors in the bar that evening and she made us all feel a lot better. Not only did most students arrive at summer school feeling like we did, but they left with solid understanding. She was absolutely right!
>
> A week later it all made sense, but looking back I cannot so easily identify what it was that made it click after so many hours of study had failed. We had good lectures, discussions with tutors, practical experiments, and discussions with other students. Something about this somehow got the quantum model into my brain.

The mode of communication is significant. For example:

- In verbal face-to-face discussions, tutorials and class-teaching environments, all channels are available; these are the best means of communicating complex information or analytical models.
- Telephone communication contains no visual cues, and it is poorer than face-to-face discussion, but it does retain intonation and tone of voice which are valuable non-verbal cues.
- Written communication contains only words and is, therefore, the most impoverished form of communication and the most difficult to understand – and the easiest to misunderstand.

This highlights how important it is to choose the right channel for the intended message. If the message is analytical or can be easily misunderstood – or if the consequences of misunderstanding are severe – then face-to-face communication is the best option.

WRITTEN (PRINTED) COMMUNICATION

The strengths of written communication are:

- It can be referred to at any time after it has been written.
- It can be skimmed or dipped into rather than read in sequence.
- It can easily be sent over long distances.
- It can be accessed by lots of people.

The weaknesses of written communication are:

- Lack of non-verbal clues.
- Lack of feedback.

Good written communication requires an effort to focus on the reader rather than the writer. Common faults are alienating the reader with curt unjustified directives, stating things that are important to the writer but not to the reader, and the use of excessively non-specific and politically correct language to avoid possible blame, rather than enhancing clarity.

These deficiencies of written communication do not affect all messages equally. It is good for factual transfer, but bad for conveying understanding of complex issues, addressing concerns, and conflict resolution. For these issues face-to-face conversation should be used whenever possible.

TELEPHONE COMMUNICATION

Telephone communication is somewhere in between face-to-face communication and written communication. However, face-to-face conversation should be used where possible, because while intonation and tone of the voice are useful non-verbal cues, there are no visual cues.

COMPUTER-MEDIATED COMMUNICATION

By computer-mediated communication we mean person-to-person communication such as email, mobile phone text-messaging or instant-messenger services of the kind provided by Yahoo, Microsoft and Research in Motion's Blackberry system.

It is easy to send out a text message or email message that you later regret! Once a message has been sent, you lose control over who reads it. It can be forwarded to any number of people or stored indefinitely, unknown and inaccessible to you, and later found by powerful search-engine software and the original message taken out of context.

> These systems are fast, with completely accurate message transmission – but humans are not. For us, more speed means less accuracy.

We cannot physically write and post an angry letter in just a few seconds, but these new channels of communication make it possible.

The computer-based media are simply bad for communicating emotion. Whatever the Sender intends, the Receiver is likely to interpret emotional content as more *negative* than intended, either seeing neutrality where positive emotion was intended, or negative where neutral was intended. As a consequence, such messages lead to greater conflict than other communication channels.

Experimental evidence shows that decisions made by groups who communicate electronically are poorer than those of groups who communicate face-to-face. And they are even worse with electronic media that are text only, compared to those with some audio or video component, or if they are non-synchronous (meaning that, like email, they do not invite an immediate response).

HANDWRITTEN COMMUNICATION

Errors in drug administration are often due to unclear handwriting, particularly of numbers and unit symbols. For example:

- When "U" is used for "unit" (especially of insulin), it can look like "0" (zero)
- When "μg" is used for "mcg" (microgram), "μ" can look like "m" (milli)

- When trailing zeros are used after a decimal point (2.0 versus 2), "2.0" can look like "20".

- When leading decimal points are used with no zero (.2 versus 0.2), ".2" can look like "2".

- In side-specific interventions (especially surgical procedures), lower case letters "l" and "r" used for denoting left and right, can look like each other.

Another risk is the use of abbreviations, such as TLAs (three-letter acronyms).

> TLAs are poorly standardised and poorly understood. They must be used with care and written in plain English unless all relevant readers will unambiguously understand what they mean.

As the NHS makes the change to electronic prescribing, another group of errors will no doubt appear. There is emerging evidence of reduced error rates, but in other safety-critical areas such as aviation, over the longer term, over-dependence on the infallibility of such systems has developed, especially in those with little experience of manual systems.

"To err is human – but to really foul things up requires a computer"

This (anonymous) principle was clearly illustrated by the radiotherapy department at a hospital in Stoke-on-Trent, as shown in the following vignette.

Vignette 7.4 Radiation dosing

Between 1982 and 1991 the radiotherapy unit in Stoke on Trent in the UK suffered from an error that caused 1045 cancer patients to receive between 5 and 35% under-dosing. An estimated 492 patients suffered earlier tumour recurrence. The error arose because prior to 1982 staff applied a correction factor to doses. In 1982 a computer system was introduced that applied this correction automatically but staff were not aware of this feature of the system, so continued to apply the correction themselves. The error only came to light when a new computer system was installed in 1991 and a discrepancy between its dosing and previous dosing was recognised.

Receiver (SMCR)

Have you ever been reading when your mind has wandered off onto other things? You reach the end of a page and realise you have not registered anything that was on it? This happens with both reading and listening. When listening, it is more likely to happen when the Receiver is preoccupied by other concerns, or is thinking about what to say next, or is looking for a gap in the speaker's flow to interrupt them (so-called gap searching). These factors are particularly important in situations of conflict or disagreement, which is why *active listening* is a prominent part of conflict-resolution strategies.

ACTIVE LISTENING

Active listening involves the Receiver asking themselves:

"What is being said here?"

If there is no clear answer, the Receiver asks for clarification. During active listening, the Receiver should make attempts to engage the Sender with positive body language and gestures that demonstrate that the Sender is being listened to. It may be necessary, if the Sender has diverted from the message, for the Receiver to acknowledge this and check that they intended to move away from the original message.

Feedback (closed-loop communication)

Feedback means that the Sender gets confirmation back from the Receiver that a message has been correctly understood. It is used synonymously with the term "closed-loop communication" because of the loop sender – channel – receiver – channel – sender. In critical communication situations, such as those common in air traffic control, read-back systems are used to confirm correct transfer of data.

In education, students are asked to consult literature and then express the concepts they read about in their own terms in essay format; the idea is to test not only their ability to write essays, but also their ability to grasp the concepts they have read.

When someone calls the emergency services to report that a building is on fire, the telephonist uses structured communication to get the essential facts about where the fire is and how many people are in the building, and always asks for a contact telephone number for the caller. This structured communication is then passed on downwards along the chain and given to the fire crews who attend the scene. The contact phone number closes the communication loop. If the fire crew need clarification or fail to understand something, the caller can be contacted.

Closed-loop communication aids accuracy in situations involving complex and critical information. It is also important in the operating-theatre environment. In simulated theatre communication situations, lack of closed-loop communications has been found to be one of the factors leading to underperformance. It now forms part of the national patient safety goal in the UK.

Specific communication situations

Serial communicating through multiple people

Serial communication through multiple people occurs when information is passed from one person to another, and then on to another. It is generally an unreliable method, but often unavoidable. For structured communication, it can be tolerably reliable; but for narrative communication, it is very unreliable. It is widely used in healthcare, however, and is one of the most frequent causes of disasters and litigation.

> **Vignette 7.5 Discharged subarachnoid haemorrhage**
>
> A 35-year-old mother presented to Accident and Emergency with a sudden headache. She was seen by a registrar. Concerned about the possibility of a subarachnoid haemorrhage they organised a CT scan. This was normal.
>
> The registrar discussed the matter with the consultant who also saw the patient. The consultant was accustomed to treating headaches and also considered the history highly suspicious of a subarachnoid haemorrhage. He suggested a lumbar puncture.
>
> The result was ambiguous, with some blood staining that could have been the result of the lumbar puncture itself rather than a haemorrhage. The consultant felt a haemorrhage had not been adequately excluded and asked the registrar to phone the neurosurgeons. The registrar rang the neurosurgical registrar and communicated a headache with a normal CT and non-diagnostic lumbar puncture. Detailed analysis of the lumbar puncture was suggested and the result implied that the blood staining was not due to subarachnoid haemorrhage.
>
> The neurosurgical registrar then told the neurosurgical consultant that a patient had been referred with headache, a normal CT and "traumatic tap" lumbar puncture. The neurosurgical consultant did not accept the patient and she was discharged from Accident and Emergency. She re-presented ten days later with a severe subarachnoid haemorrhage from which she died.
>
> The episode led to a complaint and in the course of its investigation the two consultants met. It became clear that had the concerns of the Accident and Emergency consultant been conveyed properly to the neurosurgeon he would have accepted the patient without hesitation for investigation and her life would probability have been saved.

None of the steps in the above serial communication were in themselves unreasonable. The tests relied upon were not 100% accurate (no tests are) and vital information did not get through: a senior doctor who was highly experienced in the diagnosis of headaches, felt subarachnoid haemorrhage remained a possibility despite the results. This got missed out when the story was relayed.

A number of things can be done to minimise the problems associated with serial communication.

- The most obvious it to avoid it altogether – but that is not always possible. It helps if the person at one end of the chain of a serial communication is aware of its fallibility.

- Then, if something does not seem right, they can pick up the phone and speak to the person at the other end of the chain.

In the previous vignette, the Accident and Emergency consultant remained concerned about his patient, but took no further action because he accepted the opinion of the specialists. He was unaware that his message had been distorted by serial communication, so that the very reason for the referral had been lost.

> Be careful of serial communication – know when it is occurring and how unreliable it is.
> If in doubt – bypass it.

The serial communication chain consists of a person who originates the information, a person who receives it and, in between, one or more people who pass it on. In most situations, those at either end of the chain are more senior, or have more relevant knowledge or experience than those in the middle of the chain. This leads to an important conclusion: if you are initiating a chain of serial communication, then you should structure your message rather than leaving it as purely narrative.

A useful method is to enumerate the specific points to be communicated. One structure using enumeration that might have helped in the previous vignette is as follows:

1. The patient is a young woman who has a headache and is fully conscious
(i.e. There is a lot to lose if we get it wrong.)

2. We have investigated for a subarachnoid haemorrhage with inconclusive results.

3. The Accident and Emergency consultant considers the clinical picture to be suspicious despite the test results.

Parallel communicating to multiple people

Parallel communicating means giving a message to several people at the same time. It covers both public speaking and group discussion, but it is the latter that is principally relevant to team-working. Parallel communication differs from one-to-one communication in several significant ways:

- There is a greatly reduced opportunity for feedback.
- The level of attention from individual listeners is generally lower.
- Uninterrupted speaking tends to go on for longer.
- The proportion of what is remembered and retained by listeners is variable but generally lower.
- Listeners become bored easily.

GETTING THE BEST OUT OF GROUP DISCUSSIONS

Group discussion must be done well to get the best out of a team. The primary rule is to communicate both ways with all members of the team. When addressing the team, what the speaker says should be of interest to as many members as is possible – ideally everyone. If there is an issue that is only of interest to a small minority then, if possible, it should be dealt with in a subgroup, without taking up the time of all the members.

An extreme but common, situation is where the speaker spends time addressing an issue that is of interest exclusively to him or herself! Speakers who do this find it surprisingly difficult to spot in themselves. A good way of dealing with it is to alter the group lead; in briefing situations, this means rotating the person who leads the briefing. This helps each member of the group appreciate what it is that the others need to know.

SPEAKING OUT IN GROUPS

Some people speak out in group situations and some remain quiet. These preferences can be quite extreme. Research into group communication found that the most talkative member makes 40–50% of the comments, and the second most talkative makes 25–30%, irrespective of how large the group is. A quiet group member, however, may sit in silence as they listen to an issue being discussed, about which they alone know the appropriate solution, and yet they may never say a thing. Getting quiet members to speak up is difficult, but it is important not to make matters worse. The first step is to not try to elicit anything from such an individual – give them space and pay careful attention when they do speak. Asking them a direct question in public can appear threatening and he or she will usually give a bland and non-committal answer. A more effective alternative is to make a private request for an opinion later on.

The three-point rule

The three-point rule is widely used in public speaking and group briefings. It depends on the fact that the human brain is best at assimilating just three related points. If a fourth point is made, one or more are likely to be lost. Two points have less impact. A message is presented in two ways below:

> **Version One**—"I'm giving you the task of developing a system to prevent errors in theatre. The system is to be reliable and once implemented it must remain in use in the longer term."
>
> **Version Two**—""I'm giving you the task of developing a system to prevent errors in theatre. It must work, it must work reliably, and it must work long term."

The second version has more impact, even though it has been expanded from a message with two qualifiers to a message with three qualifiers, one of which is redundant (i.e. "*It must work*"). The three-point rule works on several levels:

- When applied to our own communication it helps to clarify thoughts on what needs to be said.
- It helps make what is said more memorable.
- It helps the listener to structure a response to the message because they are immediately keyed-in to a three-point structure which can then be used mentally to formulate a response.

Organisational issues

Weak management, failure to engage or consult with staff, and interpersonal conflicts are just some of the organisational impediments to communication. Specific measures that enhance communication are:

- Clarity of the organisational structure so it is clear who should communicate to whom, while minimising serial communication.
- Effective information technology (IT) systems.
- Clearly defined roles and responsibilities for each person.
- Appropriate supervision and training of each person, so they are familiar with the organisation's lines of communication and IT services.
- Minimising physical barriers and the effects of predictable environmental noise.
- Designing buildings that ensure staff are located together, rather than in different parts of a building or on different sites.
- Reducing any distractions (e.g. background noise, poor lighting, inappropriate temperatures, out-of-date equipment and inappropriate staffing levels).
- Carrying out dedicated communication sessions (e.g. handover, briefing, debriefing, appraisals, departmental meetings, and non-operational talk time).

Several dedicated communication sessions are described overpage.

Handover

Handover between teams ensures that all members understand the common task and their role in it, and they will have the necessary information to perform their role efficiently. It also promotes cohesion on an emotional level. These two purposes are served by *time-tabled briefing* and *shift handover*. The British Medical Association booklet recommends: the following with respect to handover

- It should occur at a fixed time and place.
- There is clear leadership.
- Any new staff are introduced.
- It is done with as few distractions as possible (such as pagers and phones).
- It is done inside of working shifts.
- There are structured prompts of issues and patients to discuss.

> There are situations in which handover with special care is called for. These are:
> - During plant maintenance.
> - When safety systems have been overridden.
> - When deviation from normal working practice is in progress or recommended.
> - When the handover is from experienced staff to inexperienced staff.

Debriefing

Debriefing is discussed in detail in *Module 5*. One objective of team communication is to maintain or improve the team's performance over a period of time. This is done by the team regularly reviewing their performance and identifying areas in which it could improve. This is the role of debriefing.

There have been several attempts to introduce formal debriefing sessions into healthcare alongside briefings, but these attempts have generally failed. Debriefing is a lower priority than briefing because it has less immediate relevance. In the case of operating theatres, the tasks of different team members do not all end simultaneously, so there is no easy time to arrange a meeting when everyone is finished.

In the longer term, the teams that debrief are the best performing ones, and it is suggested that the system of "hot debriefing" is used. With this method, any issues that could be improved, or things that have gone particularly well and could be repeated, are discussed as soon as practicable after they arise.

Operational talk times

In aviation, the times of take-off and landing are busy and risky. To reduce background noise, communication in the cabin is limited to operational talk only. In healthcare the same method can be used during high-risk periods. Outside these periods, non-operational talk has a role in team dynamics and should not be prohibited.

Potential operational talk times in a clinical situation are during anaesthetic induction and intubation, preoperative checking, and times of critical decision-making.

Conclusions

Communication failures are a major cause of mistakes, complaints and litigation in healthcare. Staff should be aware of particular danger areas such as serial communication, misleading sound bites, and inadequate briefings and handovers.

Match the mode of communication to the message. Complex or messages and ones where misunderstanding would be particularly harmful should be given face-to-face. Telephone and written communications perform less well in such cases. Modern text-based instant messaging systems are prone to aggravate conflict rather than alleviate it. Perhaps the clearest message about improving communication is *think before speaking*.

Stress and Fatigue

Key points for reflection

❶ Stress is only an indirect consequence of stressors; it is a direct consequence of stressors that exceed coping resources.

❷ Ample evidence shows that stress leads to poor performance and health risks.

❸ We have little control over our own stressors but we can control:
   i. Our coping resources`
   ii. The stress we cause to others

In this module we look at work-related stress and how it affects the performance and health of staff. Stress is divided into acute and chronic forms.

Acute stress is the 'fight or flight' reaction. Its effects include fear, anger and fixation on narrow issues. Much acute stress is uncontrollable, but there are specific situations that cause acute stress such as conflict that can be managed (as can its consequences).

Chronic stress is not the same as protracted or often-repeated acute stress. Chronic stress is a consequence of cumulative demands on a person – commitments, frequent interruptions and unnecessary tasks that require an individual to work out what is needed despite poor communication. Chronic stressors are the main target for stress management.

Workplace stress

Self-report

The main tool used in stress research is self-reported stress levels. Around 20–40% of working people report stress-related health problems or stress-related sick leave. In the UK, stress is the second most common work-related health problem after musculoskeletal disorders. The current culture and politics in the UK incline towards being sympathetic to stress-related problems, and compensating for them. The problems depend on self-reporting and are generally not amenable to objective testing. They are often associated with secondary gains such as prolonged paid absence from work; in fact, the current epidemic of self-reported stress-related illness may relate to such secondary gains. When planning stress-reducing interventions, what we really want to know is their likely effect on non-self-reported measures, such as rates of sick leave and staff turnover, but data on these are minimal.

Attitudes to stress

Workplace stress is a major issue across industry because of the economic importance of sick leave and the potential for employees to seek compensation from their employers. Stress-related illness is common among healthcare staff.

Stress tolerance is known to vary widely between individuals. For example, the senior decision-makers in organisations tend to be hard-working, driven and capable. Such people often think that intolerance of stress is a sign of personal weakness or inadequacy. They are frequently tolerant of stress themselves or, if they are intolerant, they refuse to admit the fact, and tend to believe (as did US President Harry S. Truman) that people who 'cannot stand the heat should get out of the kitchen'.

This means that while senior decision-makers may understand the relationship between workplace stress and issues such as sick leave, they find it difficult to identify with the problem themselves.

The healthcare culture is characterised by the idea of personal invulnerability, led by the medical profession. Consultants in general, and surgeons in particular, are more inclined to deny that their performance is degraded by stress and fatigue than professionals in other fields.

Published research tells a different story. A body of evidence shows that healthcare workers are particularly prone to stress, and that it can be managed, and that it affects patient safety. Stress-related illness among healthcare staff is associated with significant impairment of patient care.

Stressors and resources

Stressors are the demands placed upon people, but they are not the direct cause of stress. The direct cause of stress is the demands we face that exceed our ability to cope with them. For example, having a mortgage is a stressor; having a mortgage of two thousand pounds a month a fixed stressor. It might cause someone on a high income a trivial amount of stress, but to someone on an average income it will cause considerable stress.

> The effect of stressors depends on the demand they place and the ability cope with them. The ability to cope depends on the mental, social and material support available to an individual. These are known as stress-coping *resources*, and they are generally more important than stressors.

Most surveys show that workers who are low down in an organisation's hierarchy are the most stressed. They might not have highly demanding jobs, but they have little control and this causes them stress. Deadlines in the workplace are another example of stressors; help with the task and time are both resources that reduce their effect.

Table 8.1 lists some common stressors and their associated resources. These stressors are manageable, chronic, and low level. They can be assessed and moderated, or coping resources can be provided, but they are difficult to quantify. Despite the importance of resources, much of the research ignores them because they are so difficult to measure.

Table 8.1 *Chronic stressors and associated resources*

Chronic stressors	Comments	Resources
Time pressure	■ Too much pressure gives stress; too little, causes boredom ■ Staff who control their own workload find their balance; those who do not are prone to stress or boredom ■ Time pressure reduces surgical dexterity under experimental conditions	■ Time ■ Control over workload ■ Flexibility of commitments ■ Help with tasks from others
Noise	■ Includes background noise ■ Non-operational talk during critical tasks ■ Construction and maintenance work noise	■ Freedom to avoid it ■ Ear protection ■ Operational talk times
Change	■ Affects different personalities differently ■ Stresses judging temperaments more than perceiving ones	■ Consultation about and explanation of change ■ Flexibility about change and its implementation
Distractions	■ Affects judging temperaments more than perceiving. Distracting tasks reduce surgical dexterity under experimental conditions	■ Co-workers who can deal with distractions such as phone calls while critical tasks are in progress
Not knowing what is expected of you	■ Common and easily manageable	■ Communication and briefing from co-workers
Supervisors and managers	■ Particularly autocratic or toxic leadership behaviour	■ Participation in decision making
Divided loyalties	■ Between home and work ■ Particularly relates to time pressure	■ Control over working hours ■ Control over shift patterns
Lack of control	■ Greatest workplace stressor ■ Lack of job control is associated with cardiovascular disease	■ Democratic leadership style

Life event stressors

Most research looks only at stressors. One approach to the measurement of stress, therefore, is counting life-event stressors. Life events are not chronic and cannot, in general, be modified. They are things like sitting exams, suffering a bereavement, changing jobs and getting married. The advantage of measuring these stressors is that the data can accurately and reliably be collected from subjects on their life-event history. The method can be used to investigate the effects of stress on health and performance. The best known list of life-event stressors is that of Holmes and Rahe. The 1967 version of the social readjustment rating scale is reproduced in **Table 8.2** (overpage).

This ranks a number of common life events and gives them a numerical value that is worked out relative to the stress of getting married (scores as 50). The scale allows cumulative stress over time to be calculated.

Adverse effects of stress

Behavioural effects

Behavioural responses such as irritability, hostility and apathy are often caused by stress, but the key clue that someone is over-stressed is the change in their behaviour rather than behaviour per se. New patterns of hostility, alcohol or tobacco use, apathy, absenteeism or carelessness in someone who normally does not show these traits is an indicator of serious chronic stress.

Emotional effects

As with behavioural patterns, it is the change in emotional patterns that is most suggestive of a stress reaction. Most stress-induced emotions are part of our coping resources and are positive (such as determination, concentration and pride in success), but when the stress exceeds our resources, negative emotions appear (such as cynicism, depression, anxiety and irritability).

Systemic disease effects

Holmes and Rahe's social readjustment rating scale (**Table 8.2**) was used in the 1960s to study the patterns of stress that preceded the onset of disease symptoms in groups of patients and controls. They found that the patients showed a clustering of stressors in the two years preceding the onset of their symptoms, which differed significantly from controls. Correlations between scores on the social readjustment scale and disease have been revised numerous times since the 1960s, but they always give broadly similar findings – that cumulative stress is associated with the onset of disease.

Stress has numerous associations with disease, but these may not all be because stress causes the disease. Ill health is a major stressor and any association may be because a disease causes stress rather than the other way round. Another link is that the sections of society who are most prone to ill health also tend to be those who are prone to stress, such as those with low socioeconomic status.

Mindful of these reservations, chronic stress does seem to cause a non-specific depression of defence mechanisms. It is associated with an increased risk of cardiovascular disease, but its most pronounced association is with exacerbation of an existing disease. For example, stress causes cancer to behave more aggressively (whether it has an influence on the incidence of cancer is less clear, but there is some evidence that it increases it). Numerous other diseases show this relationship with stress too:

- It is associated with worsening control of inflammatory bowel disease.
- It extends the time it takes for wounds to heal by 25%.
- It delays postoperative recovery in general, so that few surgeons will perform non-urgent surgery on patients who are highly distressed or frightened.
- It delays recovery from tuberculosis; it has long been known that patients with a positive, optimistic and cheerful outlook recover faster.
- It provokes or exacerbates both neuroses (anxiety states) and disorders of affect (depression) (the closest and best described disease associations of stress are with mental illness).
- The longstanding concepts of 'fighting off' a disease and 'dying of a broken heart' date from a time when mortal diseases characterised by a chronic balance between body defence and disease progress were common.

Table 8.2 *Holmes and Rahe's 1967 social readjustment rating scale of life events*

Life event	Life-change units
Death of a spouse	100
Divorce	73
Marital separation	65
Death of a close family member	63
Imprisonment	63
Personal injury or illness	53
GETTING MARRIED	**50**
Dismissal from work	47
Retirement	45
Marital reconciliation	45
Change in health of family member	44
Pregnancy	40
Business readjustment	39
Sexual difficulties	39
Gain of a new family member	39
Change in financial state	38
Death of a close friend	37
Change to a different line of work	36
Change in frequency of arguments	35
Major mortgage	32
Foreclosure of mortgage or loan	30
Change in responsibilities at work	29
Trouble with in-laws	29
Leaving of child from home	29
Outstanding personal achievement	28
Spouse starts or stops work	26
Begin or end school	26
Change in living conditions	25
Revision of personal habits	24
Trouble with boss	23
Change in working hours or conditions	20
Change in schools	20
Change in residence	20
Change in recreation	19
Change in church activities	19
Change in social activities	18
Minor mortgage or loan	17
Change in sleeping habits	16
Change in eating habits	15
Change in number of family reunions	15
Vacation	13
Christmas	12
Minor violation of the law	11

These relationships between organic conditions and stress only account for a minority of stress-related ill health and lost work days. The commonest manifestations of stress are symptoms that resist diagnosis on objective testing, such as tension headaches, chronic fatigue and irritable bowel syndrome, and conditions that are endemic but whose clinical manifestations are highly variable and subject to psychosomatic exacerbation, such as arthritis and spondylitis.

Cognitive function effects

Experimentally, high levels of stress have been found to impair short-term memory, decision-making, forward planning and the ability to prioritise. This effect on prioritisation is significant because it reflects a situation we all recognise, whereby stress impairs the ability to see things in proportion. Stressors often cause people to concentrate on things obsessively, so they fail to see the true importance of the stressors themselves in the fuller context and running of their lives.

THE YERKES–DODSON EXPERIMENTS

Over a hundred years ago, in 1908, Yerkes and Dodson published the results of a series of experiments. In these experiments, mice were placed in a chamber with two tunnels – a dark tunnel leading to a dead end, and a light tunnel leading to a nest. The position of the tunnels was changed at random. The experiments measured how long it took the mice to learn to go through the light tunnel. Motivation was added by giving the mice an electric shock (through wires in the floor) if they went into the dark tunnel. Two factors were varied: the size of the shock they received and the difference in grey tone (light level) between the dark and light tunnels. The results are shown in **Figure 8.1**.

When the task was easy (with the light level set at black versus white tunnel), the larger the electric shock the faster the mice learned (curve II). When the task was more difficult (with less difference between the shades of grey, an intermediate difference in curve I and slight difference in curve III) the learning was faster for intermediate shocks than for either small or large shocks. This led to the generation of the "Yerkes–Dodson law" which states that performance increases to a peak with increasing stress, then declines with further increases in stress – this effect is known as called hormesis.

The alternative model is known as the "catastrophe model". This model proposes that physiological arousal displays a mild inverted-U relationship (like that of Yerkes–Dodson) with performance when cognitive anxiety is low, but catastrophic declines in performance can occur if both physiological arousal and cognitive anxiety are high.

Yerkes–Dodson effects have been claimed for several cognitive functions, such as memory, visual perception, eye-witness recall and simulator-assessed laparoscopic surgical dexterity. The stylised graph shown in **Figure 8.2** is one that appears often in the literature, but its message remains unproven. It suggests markedly different outcomes compared to alternative theories, indicating a gradual – rather than a catastrophic – decline in performance as stress increases.

> ### What is hormesis?
> The Yerkes–Dodson curve is an example of hormesis, an effect found in pharmacology, toxicology and environmental health whereby an agent has an effect which rises with dose up to a maximum, then falls with further increases in dose, passing again through zero to become negative (like the effect of alcohol intake on the incidence of heart disease; it protects from heart attacks at low doses but causes heart disease at high doses). It has been extensively investigated in relation to ageing, with radiation, oxidative stress and food restriction, which all show hormesis in experimental conditions.

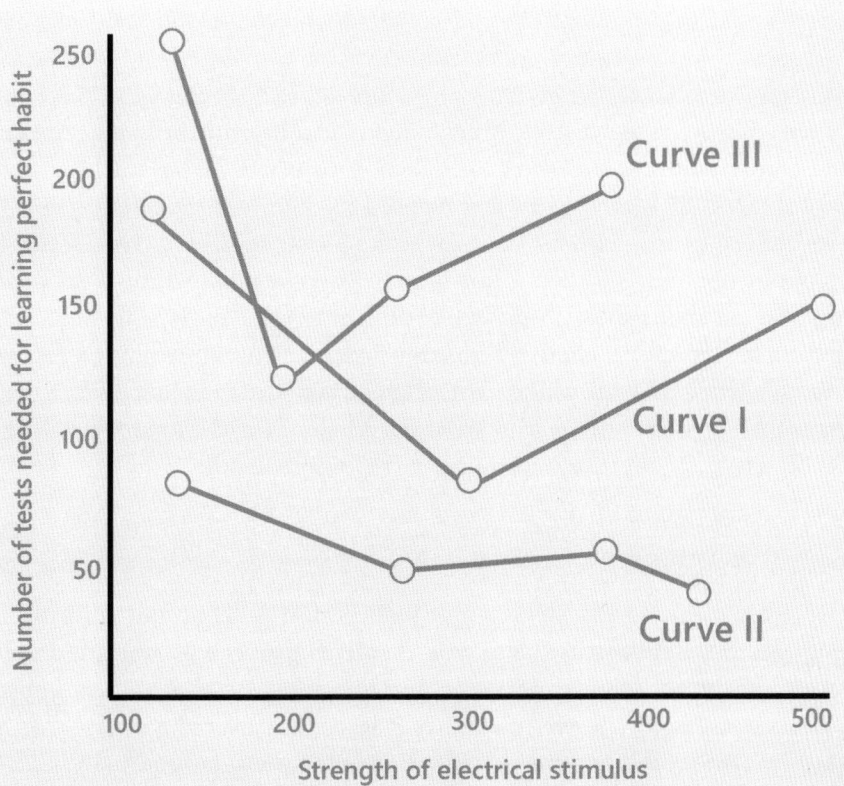

A graphic representation of strength of electrical stimulus to condition of visual discrimination and rapidity of learning. Ordinates represent value of electrical stimulus in units of stimulation; abscisae represent the number of tests given. Curve I represents the results of the experiments of Set I. Each dot indicates a value of stimulus which was used in the experiments. For example, the first dot to the left in Curve I signifies that the stimulus whose value was 125 units gave a perfect habit, in the case of the four individuals trained, with 187 tests; the second dot, that for the stimulus value of 300 units, 80 tests were necessary; and the third that for the stimulus value of 500, 155 tests. Curves II and III represent the results of mice Sets II and III, respectively.

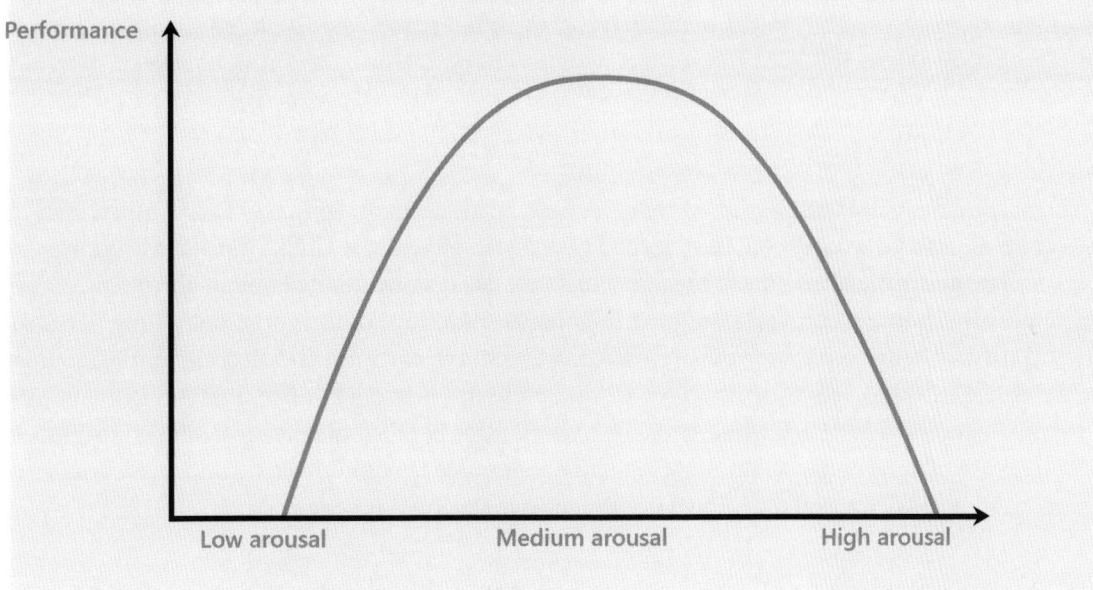

Figure 8.1 **Upper panel:** *The Yerkes–Dodson's relationship between stimulus strength and visual discrimination and learning in mice published in 1908 (curves I–III show the results of three sets of experiments; the detailed caption is reproduced from the original).* **Lower panel:** *Stylised version of the Yerkes–Dodson relationship as found in the popular psychology press (treat with caution!).*

Stress management

The Health and Safety Executive Stress Management system

The default way of managing stress is reactive; if an individual complains of being overstressed, the matter is investigated and appropriate measures are taken. Organisations have a legal obligation to manage the work-related stress their employees are exposed to. They are expected to assess stressors and, where reasonable, reduce them – rather than treat stress purely reactively. The Health and Safety Executive (HSE) has outlined a means of doing this by *risk assessment*, which involves professionally staffed studies asking workers about stress, *translation* (designing interventions to reduce stress) and *intervention* (putting them into practice). There is a close relationship between avoiding stress and serving the less worthy motives of idleness and greed, and many changes aimed at reducing stress also serve these motives. It is no surprise then that wherever workplace stress is looked for, it is found. Determining when the HSE approach can lead to cost–effective improvements requires balance!

Cultural stress management

In a cultural model of stress management, stress is not looked at in isolation but is incorporated into human factors training generally. The issues of team-work, leadership and communication all have direct bearings on levels of stress, and understanding the importance of stress adds motivation to improve performance in those same areas. While we may have little control over the stresses we personally experience, we frequently have greater control over the stresses of those around us. With appropriate team-work, leadership and communication skills we can work with those around us to reduce the stress we all experience far more effectively than anything we can achieve as lone individuals.

Conflict and conflict resolution

Conflict resolution is a major issue in healthcare, where staff must deal with violence and aggression from the public. In 1999, the NHS began a campaign of 'zero tolerance' against violence and aggression and has training material for this. Our focus is not on this, but on the issue of conflict between staff.

Causes of team conflict

Team conflicts are traditionally classified into three types: task, relationship, and process. Task conflicts involve differences of opinion about what should be done and how it should be done. Unlike the other two forms of conflict, this can be positive and beneficial, because it includes discussions about planning and policy, and is part of the process of choosing between alternative options. Relationship conflicts arise out of interpersonal animosity and are usually expressed in terms of complaints about lack of communication, unfair distribution of resources, or victimisation, but these issues are secondary to interpersonal dislike. Partly because of this tendency to use surrogates for the main issue of conflict, relationship conflicts are the most difficult to resolve. Process conflicts are disagreements about delegation and about who should do what. Unlike task conflicts, they are personalised by linkage with individual team members' skills and time usage.

Management of conflict

In a study on the performance of 57 teams of students involved in tasks relevant to their grades, researchers were able to map the teams into four groups using two dichotomies: well-performing or improving versus poor-performing or deteriorating, and high versus low team-member satisfaction. **Figure 8.2** summarises the results.

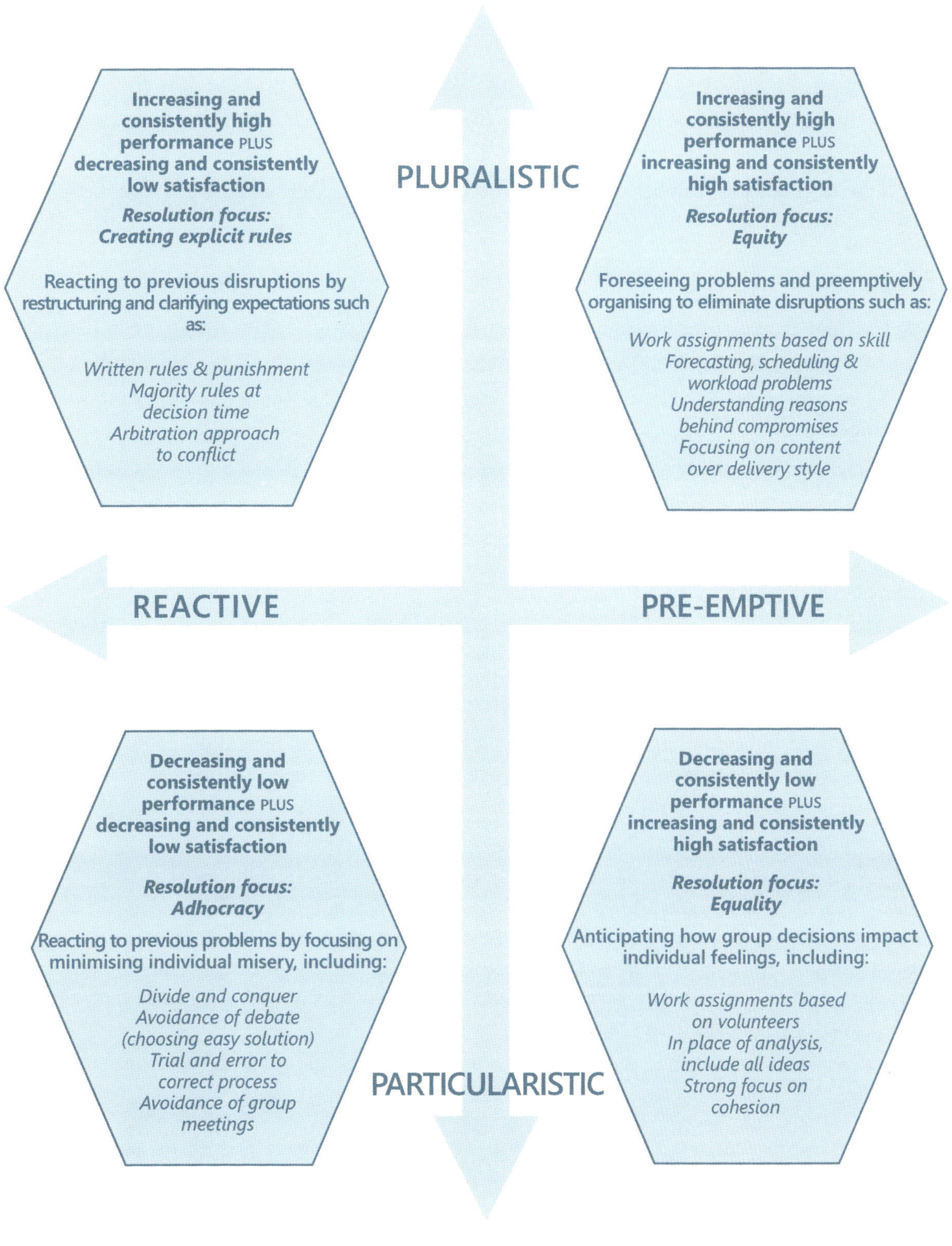

PLURALISTIC / REACTIVE

Increasing and consistently high performance PLUS **decreasing and consistently low satisfaction**

Resolution focus: Creating explicit rules

Reacting to previous disruptions by restructuring and clarifying expectations such as:

*Written rules & punishment
Majority rules at decision time
Arbitration approach to conflict*

PLURALISTIC / PRE-EMPTIVE

Increasing and consistently high performance PLUS **increasing and consistently high satisfaction**

Resolution focus: Equity

Foreseeing problems and preemptively organising to eliminate disruptions such as:

*Work assignments based on skill
Forecasting, scheduling & workload problems
Understanding reasons behind compromises
Focusing on content over delivery style*

PARTICULARISTIC / REACTIVE

Decreasing and consistently low performance PLUS **decreasing and consistently low satisfaction**

Resolution focus: Adhocracy

Reacting to previous problems by focusing on minimising individual misery, including:

*Divide and conquer
Avoidance of debate (choosing easy solution)
Trial and error to correct process
Avoidance of group meetings*

PARTICULARISTIC / PRE-EMPTIVE

Decreasing and consistently low performance PLUS **increasing and consistently high satisfaction**

Resolution focus: Equality

Anticipating how group decisions impact individual feelings, including:

*Work assignments based on volunteers
In place of analysis, include all ideas
Strong focus on cohesion*

Figure 8.2 *Matrix of different conflict management strategies (pluralistic, particularistic, reactive and pre-emptive) on performance and satisfaction in teams.*

From this study emerged three strategies for conflict management that were consistently associated with high team-member satisfaction and good or improving performance of the team as a whole. These were:

- Focusing on the issues rather than the way in which they are presented by team members.
- Explicitly discussing the reasons behind decisions made in allocating tasks to team members and their acceptance of them.
- Allocating tasks to members who have the relevant expertise, rather than by other methods (such as volunteering, default, convenience or willingness).

There are numerous conflict resolution methods with different names, but common key points are:

- If a conflict arises within a team it is almost always better to resolve it within the team rather than recourse to external arbitration or authority.
- Agree with the other side what the contentious issue is so that you are not debating over a misunderstanding.
- Separate relationships between the people from the issues and prioritise good relationships
- Listen first – talk second!

Anger management

Conflict resolution is concerned with managing disagreement with others, while anger management is about managing ourselves. People vary in their susceptibility to anger, from placid, docile individuals to irritable, quick-tempered ones. At the angry end of the spectrum this behaviour pattern can be detrimental to an individual, and the group in which they work. Around 5% of people have a problem with anger. Treatments for anger are forms of psychotherapy.

- **Cognitive behavioural therapy (CBT)**

CBT for destructive anger explores provoking factors and how to respond to them, the self-sustaining effect of thoughts and behavioural reinforcement in anger escalation, and the consequences of a person's anger on themselves and those around them. It may be administered as group therapy to create an environment where individuals can openly discuss their problems with others who have personal knowledge of them and without judgement from those unaffected by destructive anger.

- **Psychodynamic therapy**

This form of therapy is from the Freudian school of psychoanalysis; it explores putative underlying primal motivations and influences originating from repressed memories. The theory is that by bringing these things to conscious recognition, anger can be reduced.

Programmes for anger management involve either an intensive course of therapy over a few days, or repeated sessions over weeks or months, with detection and treatment of relapses if disruptive behaviour should return.

The UK Department of Health runs a Practitioner Health Programme for medical staff in the London area that addresses anger, but it is mainly concerned with substance abuse. The Cardiff Deanery runs a programme for doctors with behavioural problems, mainly anger and aggression related.

A common fallacy in anger management is the *hydraulic theory* that angry emotions are like a fluid under pressure that must be let out or they will lead to ill health because they are 'bottled up'. Experimental results show this to be false. Expressing anger and 'taking it out' on inanimate objects by doing acts of violence to them, or seeking 'outlets' for anger (like combat sports), all promote higher levels of anger and aggression; they also impair self-control and delay resolution in anger-provoking situations.

Post-traumatic stress disorder

Post-traumatic stress disorder (PTSD) occurs after a person has witnessed a highly stressful event (stressor) that poses a risk to life or injury to themselves or to others. It is estimated that 50% of the people in Western countries experience an event sufficient to trigger PTSD in their lifetime, but the proportion of healthcare workers is higher. Of those who experience such an event, 10–20% develop the condition. PTSD can be incapacitating and often delays or prevents a return to work. Normal responses to severe stressors include:

- Reminders of the events, e.g. flashbacks, intrusive thoughts, nightmares.
- Excitation, e.g. insomnia, agitation, irritability, anger.
- Inactivation, e.g. avoidance, withdrawal, confusion, depression.

These reactions resolve within one month of the stressful event occurring in the normal population. In PTSD, however, they persist beyond one month, for acute PTSD, and beyond three months, for chronic PTSD, or they reappear after an interval of normal recovery in delayed-onset PTSD (**Figure 8.3**).

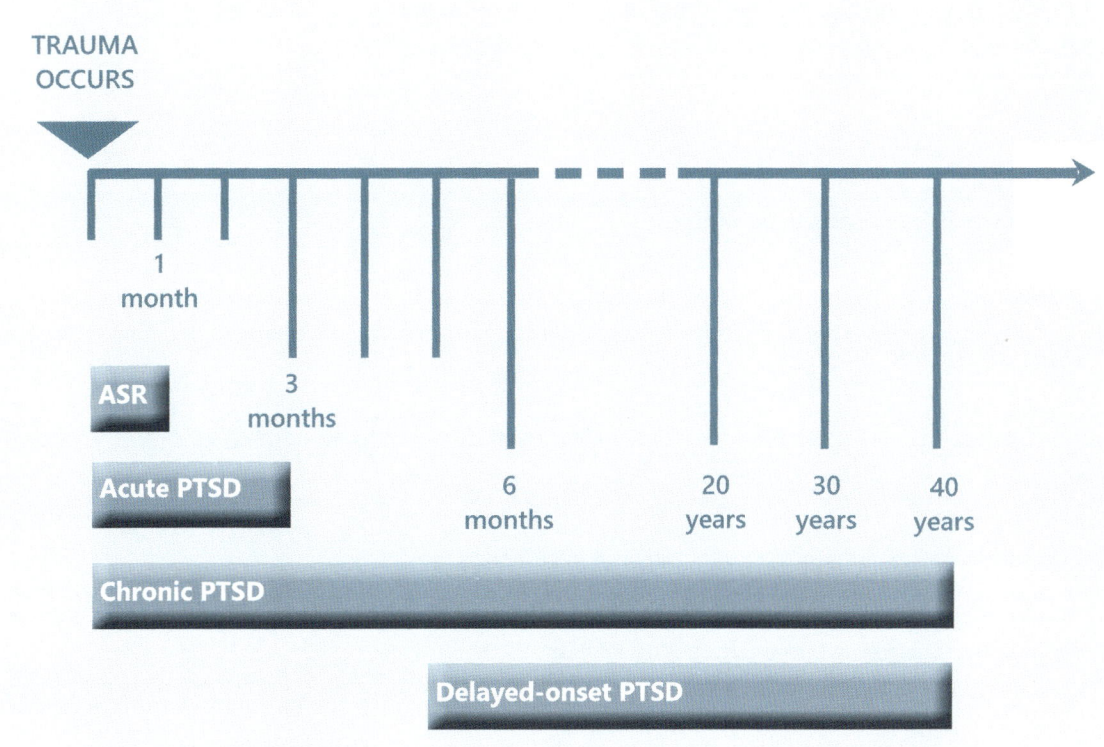

Figure 8.3 *Typical PTSD reactions to trauma at different times after an initial trauma (ASR = (normal) acute stress reaction; PTSD = post-traumatic stress disorder).*

Previously, debriefing was advised as a preventative measure after severe psychological trauma, but this *increased* the risk of PTSD! Normal recovery involves a progressive decline in the memory of and attention given to the stressful event. It is impeded by re-visiting the event in debriefing. Both treatment and prevention are aimed at social support and avoidance of memory triggers.

There are three Ps to avoid
(from Zohar et al. CNS Spectrums, 2009; 14(Suppl. 1): 44–51)

Pathologising
(symptoms within a month of the events are a normal response.)

Psychologising
(work through the issues in debriefing or group therapy)

Pharmacologising
(treating with anxiolytic drugs.)

Fatigue

Lack of sleep causes more road accidents than drugs and alcohol together. Medics' duty-hours have been reduced over the last twenty years, but surveys conducted in the 1990s report substantial rates of tiredness-related mistakes made by doctors, many of which have been fatal.

Sleepiness and sleep deprivation

Sleepiness can be measured in two ways:

- The multiple sleep latency test: this measures how long it takes someone to fall asleep.
- The pupillographic sleepiness test: this measures the fluctuations in pupil diameter that occur when we are tired.

Both measures have been used to show that healthcare staff are often moderately or severely sleepy when at work.

Sleepiness has detrimental effects on a range of performances:

- **Motor skills**—Loss of two hours sleep in one night produces impairment in motor performance equivalent to drinking two or three pints of beer.
- **Communication**— Studies observing the performance of teams engaged in prolonged tasks find that the clarity and frequency of communication declines with increasing fatigue.
- **Social**—Fatigue leads to impatience, irritability and lack of courtesy.
- **Decision making**—Impaired decision-making has been reported for people who drive or play sports, and in those in healthcare and aviation.

The amount of sleep deprivation a person can tolerate without becoming significantly sleepy at work is also dependent on other "tiring" factors, such as extremes of temperature, stress, noise, vibration, and how boring a task is. Sleep deprivation has a cumulative effect on performance, but restoration to normality is not sensitive to the *amount* – it only takes one night's good sleep to fully recover, however much sleep deprivation there has been.

Circadian rhythms

Circadian rhythms are the body's daily physiological rhythms of blood pressure, temperature and wakefulness. These rhythms run in time with the light–dark cycle of day and night and when that changes (due to jet lag, perhaps), the rhythms become 'entrained' to the new hours, adjusting themselves at a rate of about one hour per day.

The circadian rhythm is governed not by the conscious visual pathways involving rods and cones, but by light-sensitive retinal ganglion cells. These do not have the same adaption qualities as rods and cones of the retina, and most artificial evening and night-time lighting is not intense enough to fool them into entraining the circadian rhythm. Full-time nightshift workers do not usually adapt their circadian rhythm successfully.

The endogenous circadian rhythm that occurs when subjects are denied any clues about the time of day is exactly twenty-four hours long. Misinformation dating from early studies is still quoted which suggests that endogenous circadian rhythms are variable in length, with an average of around twenty-five hours.

Shifts and jet lag

Shift changes are most disruptive of sleep if they result in sleep deprivation.

> Changing from an early shift to a late shift results in tiredness during the shift, and sleep when it is over. Changing from late to early results in a lack of tiredness at the end of a shift, and difficulty sleeping, so sleep deprivation occurs before the start of the next shift.
>
> Jetlag, for the same amount of time, has less effect on tiredness if a person is travelling east rather than west – for the same reason.
>
> *This is why shifts should go 'early late night early' rather than 'early night late early'. It takes twenty-four hours to adjust to every hour's difference in sleep pattern.*

Shift work is inevitable in healthcare and there is no ideal arrangement. Current evidence suggests that the most effective option is for people to be on a particular shift for a prolonged period, rather than change shifts often. Irrespective of the shift, only a minority of workers show circadian adjustment. Advancing age increases the tiring effects of both jetlag and shift working.

SLEEP HYGIENE

To minimise sleepiness the most should be made of opportunities to sleep in the form of sleep hygiene, rest breaks and napping. Shift workers who are required to sleep during the day need extra protection from sleep disturbance due to noise and light. Opaque and closely-fitting window blinds should be used, and other occupants of the building should be informed to minimise any disturbance.

NIGHT-TIME WORKING

Nocturnal surgery has worse results than day-time surgery. Out-of-hours operations are done because of a clinical urgency and much of the extra morbidity and mortality is no doubt explained by case selection. It is not possible to separate the effects of staff tiredness from this. In other industries, case selection effects do not occur but a nocturnal safety difference is still apparent.

There is little doubt that lower team performance contributes to the poorer results of treatments given at night. To balance this disadvantage, interventions should only be undertaken at night if the expected disease progress over the hours until morning is thought to be more injurious than the extra nocturnal risk. The nocturnal risk is greatest for long or complex procedures.

Inexperienced staff tend to underestimate available time and have less reserves of skill to compensate for lowered performance at night. The often-contentious issue of what operating theatre teams should do at night is best decided with direct involvement of senior staff.

Night-workers who are required to be vigilant, such as those on look-out or monitoring safety equipment, clearly should not 'sleep on the job'. In healthcare there are large numbers of nightshift workers who do not have this role, but they are on standby to do often complicated tasks. Allowing such individuals to take naps improves their performance.

Fatigue from chronic stress

A second form of fatigue is related to cumulative chronic stress. The theory is that over time the stresses of the workplace cause a form of fatigue that leads to demotivation, 'burnout', apathy about performance, and disillusionment. This form of fatigue, if it exists (which is not certain) differs from tiredness in that it is not relieved by sleep. The theory is that it is relieved by a vacation or change of scene, as in 'a changes as good as a rest'. In contrast to tiredness and sleep deprivation, the research base behind this theory is minimal.

Conclusions

Workplace stress is an often elusive but ubiquitous and important health-related issue. Some stress is inevitable, but much of it, particularly as it affects staff working lower down in command hierarchies, is avoidable – as is the ill-health, loss of work, and staff turnover that go with it. Some specific approaches to stress management are not without controversy, but the general awareness and application of human performance and limitations has the beneficial side-effect of stress reduction.

Index

A

A-type personality, 40
abbreviations (use in communication), 76, 85
abdominal surgery, 28, 80
ability model (Mayer's), 71
absenteeism (stress related), 96
accepted practice (adherence to), 32
accident and emergency (A&E), 17, 19, 22, 37, 88
accident prevention, 97
active listening, 88
acute stress, 93
adaptive decision-making, 17
administrative staff (NHS), 54, 69
administrator (personality type), 43
adrenaline, 37, 60
adverse events (serious), 75
advocate (personality type), 43
affect disorder, 96
affected persona, 42
aggression
    dealing with, 100
    in doctors, 102, 103
    in teams, 55, 64, 65, 68
agreeableness, 41
airway compromise, 17, 18, 23, 30
alert (PACE), 37, 77
alienation (groups), 68
anaesthesia, 5, 36
Anaesthetists' Non-Technical Skills for Surgeons (ANTS), 58
analytic thinking, 1, 4, 5–7, 12, 20
anchoring (heuristic), 3
anger management, 102–103
apparatchik, 68
appendicitis, 28
appreciation (within teams), 55
architect personality type, 43

arousal and performance (under stress), 98, 99
arteries, 35, 80
artisan (personality), 40, 43, 46, 47–48, 49, 70
Asch, Solomon, 35
assessment step (SA), 15, 16, 21, 26, 29, 79
asthma, 22
authority
    authority gradient, 36, 37
    and personality type, 46, 47, 50
    in teams, 70, 102
autocratic leadership, 64, 68, 74, 95
automatic thinking
    cognitive processing, 2–5, 6, 7, 9, 12
    decision making, 20, 26
availability (heuristic), 3
aviation industry and incidents
    communication, 85, 90
    situation awareness, 34, 35
    stress and fatigue, 104
    team working, 52, 57, 61

B

B-type personality, 40
bandwagon effect, 35
bank-wiring room experiment, 54
bureaucracy (professional), 69
behaviour. *see also* aggression; emotions; leadership; personality types
    change in, 96
    displacement activities, 32
    egocentric, 65
    psychodynamic theory, 8–10
    stress, 42, 95, 96
Belbin Team Inventory, 55
Berne, Eric, 62

Index

bias
    cognitive, 1, 2, 3
    confirmation, 31, 33
Big Five personality traits (OCEAN), 40–41, 50
bile (temperament), 39
blame (in leadership), 72
blame bite, 81
bleeding (patient), 1, 17, 19, 21
blood potassium levels, 19, 20
blood pressure, 31, 32, 33, 80
blood sugar levels, 19, 20
Boeing airplane incidents, 23
brain injury and damage
    behaviour problems, 24
    brain tumour, 31
    intraoperative, 19, 31
    memory, 11, 13
    penetrating injury, 12
briefing (staff and teams), 33, 56, 72, 88, 89, 90. see also debriefing
Bristol Heart Scandal (Kennedy Report), 53
buy-in (team motivation), 54, 55, 72

C

cancer (patient), 28, 77, 85, 96
capriciousness, 68
cardiac arrest, 22
cardiovascular disease, 95, 96
case studies as evidence, 50
challenge (PACE), 37, 77
champion (personality), 43
change
    attitudes to, 44, 47, 54
    in leadership, 69, 70
    policy change, 24
    shift working, 105
    situation awareness, 34
    as stressor, 95, 97
chemotherapy, 61
chest drain, 17
cholecystectomy, 1
choleric temperament, 39, 40, 48
chronic stress, 13, 93, 95, 96, 106
circadian rhythms, 105
closed-loop communication, 86
co-amoxiclav, 5, 7
coercive power, 67

cognitive behavioural therapy (CBT), 102
cognitive bias, 1, 2, 3
cognitive processing
    analytic, 5–7
    automatic, 2–5
    decision-making, 12
    dual-process model, 1–2
    emotion, 12–13
    evolutionary aspects, 2, 3, 8
    unconscious, 8–12
command pyramids, 69
command structure (organisational), 69
commission (errors of), 4
commonality of purpose, 72
communication
    authority gradients, 36
    channels of, 84
    closed loop and feedback, 86
    in groups, 88=89
    in organisations, 89–90
    parallel, 88–89
    roadblocks, 76–77
    serial, 86–88
    situation awareness, 36–37
    theory, 75–86
competency (leadership), 73
completer–finisher (team member), 55
composer (personality), 43
comprehension (situation awareness), 34
computers, 84, 85
confirmation (heuristic), 3
confirmation bias, 31, 33
conflict
    active listening, 86
    management, 100
    resolution, 100, 102
    within teams, 51, 102
conformity experiments, 35
confusion (situation awareness), 32
conscientious (personality), 41
conscious thought, 1, 5, 8, 9, 11
consciousness, 6, 8, 9, 10
conservator (personality), 43
constructive motivation, 54
control (and stress), 93, 95, 100
coordinator (personality), 43, 55
coronary artery disease, 40
counsellor (personality), 43

crafter (personality), 43
creativity (team), 21, 55, 73
credibility (leadership), 69, 71–72
Crohn's disease, 28, 33
cultural stress management, 100
cytosine administration, 61

D

debriefing, 56, 90, 104. *see also* briefings
decision-making
    adaptive*, 17
    analytic, 15–20
    automatic, 22–24
    clinical scenarios, 17, 19, 20, 22, 23
    groups and teams, 25–26, 52, 57
    leadership, 65, 66, 68, 73
    rule-based, 20–21, 23
    somatic marker hypothesis, 24
    steps of, 25–26
    stress and fatigue, 95, 98, 104
    unconscious, 24–25
delegation of tasks. see tasks
democratic leadership, 64, 65, 68, 73
demotivation, 55, 106
disease (stress-related), 96
displacement activities, 32
display (leadership), 36
distraction (stressor), 89, 90, 95
divided loyalty, 95
dominant attitude and function, 42
drug administration and errors, 5, 28, 61–62, 81, 84. see also individual drug names
dual-process model, 1–2

E

ego, 9
egocentric behaviour, 65
emergency (PACE), 37, 77
emergency services, 56, 86
emergency situations (clinical), 5, 17, 19, 22, 34, 87
emotions
    in communication, 77, 82, 84
    emotional intelligence, 71
    emotional support, 66
    personality type, 41, 45, 48
    stress situations, 96, 103
Endsley's model, 34
engineer (personality), 43
entertainer (personality), 43
epinephrine. *see* adrenalin
errors. *see also* drug administration and errors; threats
    clerical, 4
    communication, 36, 75, 81, 84, 85, 89
    management of, 58–62
    shift takeover, 33
    surgical, 28–29, 57
    team errors, 52
    thinking systems, 2, 4, 7
evidence base (personality studies), 50
evolution of cognition, 2, 3, 8
experience
    in communication, 76, 80, 90
    decision making, 16, 22, 24
    in leadership, 65, 70
    situation awareness, 27, 29
    thinking systems, 7
extroversion, 42, 45, 50. *see also* introversion
eye surgery, 28, 29, 33

F

fatigue and tiredness
    chronic stress, 106
    circadian rhythms, 105
    cognitive effects, 4, 7, 31, 104
    communication skills, 104
    definitions, 4
    jet-lag, 105
    motor skills, 104
    shiftwork and night-working, 105
    sleep, 104, 105
    social aspects, 104
feedback
    in communication, 76, 79, 86
    team performance, 58
feeling personality, 42, 43, 45, 79
feelings (gut), 12, 24, 33
field-marshall (personality), 43
Five Factor Model (OCEAN), 40–41, 50
Five-Factor Personality Inventory (Neo), 41
fixation (of thinking), 6, 27, 30–31, 32, 33
follower maturity, 67

Index

following orders, 73
Freud, Sigmund, 8–9, 10, 102

G

Gage, Phineas, 12
Galen, 39, 45, 46, 47, 48
Galton, Frances, 63
gap searching (communication), 86
Gimli glider incident, 23
glucose levels, 19–20
groups. see also team-working
    alienation, 68
    decision-making, 25–26
    definition, 51
    error management, 58–62
    group working, 51–53
    leadership, 65, 68
    motivation, 55–57
    option checks, 26
    responsibility, 73
    speaking out in, 88
    team approach, 53–54
    training systems, 57–58
guardian (personality), 40, 43, 46–48, 70
gut feelings, 12, 24, 33

H

haemorrhage (patient), 31, 87, 88
handover (teams), 89, 90
handwritten communication, 84
healer (personality), 43
heart disease, 40, 98
heart surgery, 23, 53
Hersey–Blanchard model, 66
heuristics, 2, 3, 12, 24
hippocampus, 13
Hippocrates, 39
Hogan Personal Inventory (HPI), 41
Holmes and Rahe readjustment scale, 97
hormesis, 98
humour (leadership), 57, 73
humours (temperaments), 39
hypnosis, 8
hypotheses in SA checks, 29

I

id, 9
idealist (personality), 40, 43, 46, 48–49, 70
iliac artery, 80
immunosuppressant treatment, 28
implementer (team member), 55
implicit knowledge, 11, 24
implicit memory, 11
INCH (I Need Clarity Here), 37
inexperience. see experience
inflexible autocrat, 68
influenza pandemic, 13
inspector (personality), 43, 54
insulin administration, 19–20
intelligence, 7, 47, 71
interference (communication), 75
intrathecal drug administration, 61
intravenous drug administration, 5, 30, 61, 62
introversion, 42, 43, 45, 50
intubation (airway), 5, 17–19, 30, 78, 81
intuition, 42, 46
intuitive (personality), 43, 44, 45, 46, 48
inventor (personality), 43
inverse apparatchik, 68
irrational perceiving, 42
irritability, 96, 103, 104

J

jet lag, 105
judging (personality), 42, 43–44, 45, 95
Jowett, Wayne, 61
Jung, Carl, 41
Jungian personality systems, 41–42, 45, 49–50.
    see also Myers–Briggs Type Indicator (MTBI)
junior staff. see also experience
    clinical scenarios, 22, 57
    communication, 36, 82
    delegation of tasks, 72
    situation awareness, 7
    team working, 56, 57, 60
    uncertainty, 32

K

Keirsey Temperament Sorter (KTS), 43–49, 50
Kennedy Report, 53

kidney disease, 19, 35
Kimmel, Admiral, 13

L

laboratory studies as evidence, 50
laissez-faire leadership, 64, 65
laparotomy, 25
laryngoscopy, 17
leaders
    aggression, 68
    authoritarian, 64, 65, 74
    autocratic, 74
    blame (use of), 71
    communication, 36
    credibility, 70–71, 72
    decision-making, 68
    democratic, 64, 65, 68, 69, 73, 74, 95
    effective, 67, 71–73, 74
    humour (use of), 72
    intelligence, 71
    laissez-faire, 64
    in the NHS, 73–74
    relationship-driven, 66
    responsibility, 72
    situation awareness, 26, 34
    task driven, 66
    toxic, 68
    visibility of, 72
leadership
    apparatchik, 68
    buy-in (team motivation), 71
    command structure, 69
    commonality of purpose, 71
    competency framework, 73–74
    control, 95
    definition, 69
    error management, 58
    by example, 71
    groups and teams, 51, 57, 65, 71, 72
    motivation, 71
    positive reinforcement, 71
    and power, 69–70
    shared, 73
    situational models, 65–68
    and stress, 95, 100
    style and traits, 6, 64–65, 73
    training, 71–72, 73
    transactional and transformational, 67
leading questions, 32, 33, 57, 77
Lewin, Kurt, 64, 65, 68
life events (stressors), 95, 97
lignocaine administration, 37
listening (active), 86
lost car (vignette), 27, 33
loyalty (divided), 95
lumbar puncture, 61, 62, 87

M

Machiavelli, Niccolo, 63
management organisation, 89
mastermind (personality), 43
maturity (follower), 66, 67
Mayer–Salovey–Caruso Emotional Intelligence Test (MSCEIT), 71
mechanistic messages, 77, 78
Medical Leadership Competency Framework (MLCF), 73–74
melancholic temperament, 39, 40, 46
melanoma, 28
memory
    explicit, 11
    implicit, 11
    short-term, 77, 98
    and stress, 13
    triggers, 104
    working, 2, 24
    Yerkes–Dodson law, 98
mentor (personality), 43, 55
messages (communication)
    emotions, 84
    mechanistic, 77
    narrative, 79
    overload, 77
    structured, 78, 79
    subliminal, 10
    transformational, 77
military environment and incidents, 69
Mintzberg, Henry, 69
mitigation of errors, 60, 62
motivation (team), 54, 58, 68, 72
motor skills, 104
multidisciplinary teams, 26, 69, 74

Index

Myers–Briggs Type Indicator (MTBI), 42, 45, 46, 49, 50

N

narrative messages, 79–81, 86
National Health Service. *see* NHS (UK)
Neo-Five Factor Personality Inventory (Neo-PI), 41
nephrectomy, 35
neuroticism, 41
NHS (UK)
    command structure, 69
    communication failure, 75
    competency framework, 73–74
    conflict resolution, 100
    leadership, 69, 73–74
    prescription errors, 85
    team working, 52, 54
night-time working, 105, 106. *see also* shift working
noise
    interference in communication, 75
    and stress, 89, 90, 95, 104, 105
non-tautological prediction, 50
Non-Technical Skills for Surgeons (NOTTS), 57
Non-Technical Skills (NOTECHS), 58

O

OCEAN (personality traits), 40–41, 50
omission (errors or), 3, 4, 33
openness, 41
operational talk times, 89, 90, 95
operator (personality), 43
option checking, 17, 26
Oxford NOTECHS (ON), 58

P

PACE (decision-making), 37, 77
paediatric surgery, 28, 53
parallel communication, 88
participating-type leadership, 66
particularist strategies (conflict resolution), 101
pattern recognition, 2, 3, 5, 7, 11
peer (social) pressure, 69

perceiving (personality), 42, 43, 44, 45, 97
perception
    conscious, 9
    situation awareness, 34
    subliminal, 9
perceptual defence, 10
performance
    cognitive, 11, 24
    and fatigue, 104, 106
    feedback, 54
    group, 25, 52, 56, 65, 67, 86, 106
    and stress, 94, 98–99, 101
performer (personality), 43
personality tests, 41, 50
personality types. *see also* individual personality types; leaders
    A and B, 40
    five factors (OCEAN), 40
    horoscope effect, 50
    Jungian models, 41–42, 49–50
    Keirsey Temperament Sorter (KTS), 44–49
    Myers–Briggs (MBTI), 42–43, 45, 46
phlegmatic temperament, 39, 40
plant (team member), 55
pluralistic strategies (conflict resolution), 101
pneumothorax, 17
political motivation, 54
positive reinforcement, 72
post-traumatic stress disorder (PTSD), 103–104
potassium levels, 19, 20
power (personal), 67, 69–70
preconsciousness, 8
preemptive strategies (conflict resolution), 101
pregnancy, 97
premature closing (heuristic), 3
prescription errors. *see* drug administration and errors
probe (situation awareness), 37, 77
process conflicts, 100
process improvement (teams), 56, 58
productivity, 53, 73. *see also* performance
professional bureaucracy, 69
project and decide (decision-making), 15, 18, 19, 26
promoter (personality), 43
provider (personality), 43
psychodynamic theory, 8–9, 10
psychodynamic therapy, 102
psychosomatic illness, 9, 98
pupillographic sleepiness test, 104

Q

questionnaires as evidence, 50
questions (leading), 32, 33, 57, 77

R

radiation dose, 85, 98
rail incidents, 12, 20, 21
rational judging, 35, 42
rational perceiving, 42
rational personality type, 43, 46, 48–49, 70
rationality, 33, 82
eactive strategies (conflict resolution), 101
receiver (communication), 75–76, 77, 79, 81, 84, 85–86
recognition-primed decisions, 22
reinforcement (behavioural), 72, 102
renal artery, 80
representative (heuristic), 3
resource investigator (team member), 55
responsibility (personal), 63, 66, 68, 73
roadblocks to communication, 76–77
rule-based decisions, 2, 20–21, 23–24
rules of thumb, 2. *see also* heuristics

S

Salovey and Mayer Ability Model, 71
sanguine temperament, 39, 40, 47
satisfaction
    patient, 52
    team, 39, 54, 100–101
SBAR (situation–background–assessment–recommendation), 79
self-motivation, 71
self-reported stress, 93
selling-type leadership, 66
sensing (personality), 42, 43, 44, 45–46, 48, 50
serial communication, 86–88
serious adverse events (SAEs), 75
shaper (team member), 55
shared leadership, 73
shift working, 56, 90, 95, 105, 106. *see also* night-time working
shipping incidents, 13, 33
situation awareness (SA). *see also* PACE
    accepted practice, 32
    authority gradients, 36
    automatic decisions, 24
    briefings, 56
    clinical scenarios, 28, 29, 31, 35
    communication issues, 33, 36–37
    conflicting information, 32
    conformity experiments, 35
    fixation, 30, 32
    leading questions, 32
    levels of, 34
    SA checks, 16, 20, 30, 32, 33
    team takeover, 32
    team working, 32, 34–35, 57
    thinking systems, 7
    triggers, 15, 29, 31, 32
    uncertainty, 32
    unease, 32
sleep. *see also* fatigue and tiredness; night-time working
    habits, 97
    hygiene, 105
    lack of, 4, 104, 105
    sleep latency test, 104
    sleepiness, 104
    and stress, 106
SMCR (communication), 75, 76–85
somatic marker hypothesis, 12, 13, 24
sound bites, 81–82
specialist (team member), 55
stress
    acute, 93
    adverse effects, 96–99
    attitudes to, 94
    chronic, 13, 93, 95, 96, 106
    and conflict, 100–102
    and fatigue, 4, 104–106
    groups, 65
    hormesis, 97, 98
    management, 100, 102–103
    and performance, 98–99, 104
    personality types, 45
    post-traumatic, 103–104
    resources, 94–96
    self-reported, 93
    sleep deprivation, 4, 104–106
    stressors and life events, 8, 94–96, 97
    subliminal messages, 10
    thinking systems, 7, 20

Index

workplace, 93–94, 105–106
Yerkes–Dodson law, 98–99
structured messages, 78–80
subarachnoid haemorrhage, 87–88
subliminal perception, 9
subliminal psychodynamic activation, 10
substitution errors, 3, 4, 5
superego, 9
supervisor (personality), 43
supervisors (management), 73, 95
Sutton's slip (heuristic), 3
Swinburne University Emotional Intelligence Test (SUEIT), 71
Swiss Cheese Model, 58–59
system 1 and 2 thinking, 2, 6, 7. *see also* analytic cognition; automatic cognition
systemic disease (stress related), 96

T

tachistoscope, 9
tacit knowledge, 2
task-driven leaders, 66
tasks
    allocation and delegation, 39, 55, 64, 72
    fixation, 32
    maturity of team members, 66
    multitasking, 3, 44
tautological prediction, 50
teacher (personality), 43
team-working. *see also* groups
    appreciation and motivation, 54, 55
    bank-wiring room experiment, 54
    Belbin Team Inventory, 55
    benefits of, 52
    briefings, 56
    error and threat management, 58–61
    function, 56
    in the NHS, 52
    process improvement, 56
    skill deployment and development, 55, 56
    team approach, 53
    time issues, 56
    training, 57
    traits and roles, 57
    versus groups, 51
technical motivation, 54

telling-type leaders, 66
temperament, 40, 46–49, 95. *see also* Keirsey Temperament Sorter (KTS); personality types
thinking personality type, 7, 42, 43, 45, 70
thinking systems, 2, 6, 7. *see also* analytic thinking; automatic thinking; cognitive processing
thiopentone administration, 5, 7
threat and error management, 58, 59–61
three-letter acronyms (TLAs), 85
three-point rule (of speaking), 89
time
    operational talk time, 89, 90, 95
    stressors and resources, 94, 95
    time pressure, 7, 16, 20, 95
    use of, 56
time-tabled briefing, 90
tiredness. *see* fatigue and tiredness
toxic leaders, 65, 68, 95
training
    leadership, 69, 70, 71–72
    teams, 52, 57
Trait Emotional Intelligence Questionnaire (TEIQue), 71
trait theory, 63
traits (personality), 39, 45, 57, 63
transactional leadership, 67
transactional model, 67
transformational leadership, 67
transformational messages, 77, 78, 79, 81
transition (thinking systems), 6, 7
trap (errors), 59, 60, 61, 62
triggers (decision making), 6, 15, 16, 29–30
Turkey Creek rail incident, 20

U

unconscious mind, 24–25, 33
USS Montana incident, 33

V

vincristine administration, 61
visibility (leadership), 73
vision (in leaders), 51, 67, 74
visual system, 11

W

Western Electric Company, 53
whistle-blowers, 53
workplace stress, 83–94
written communications, 83–85
wrong diagnosis, 27, 28, 32
wrong-side surgery, 28, 33, 35, 57

Y

Yerkes–Dodson law, 98–99